Breast Cancer:
start here...

*Everything You Need to Know
About Integrative Health for
the Newly Diagnosed*

By Breast Cancer Survivor Julie A. Buckley, MD
and Reconstructive Surgeon Ankit Desai, MD

Our purpose in writing *Breast Cancer: Start Here* is to provide you with information that will empower you and your physician to make better healthcare decisions for you. The content of this book cannot replace a physician's opinion and is not intended to be used to make a diagnosis or to recommend a treatment. We recommend you use this information as you consult with your physician with respect to your medical history and unique circumstances.

Cover art by Sally Eckhoff
Interior design by Typeflow
Interior Illustrations by Sally Eckhoff

Produced in the USA

ISBN 978-1-62134-073-7

For my many Sisters.

May there be healing, and may there be many who never join our sisterhood because they find Health before breast cancer finds them!

And for my parents.

Both of whom taught me by example to approach cancer with grace, dignity, determination, and ferocity.

Julie

For all my courageous patients,
who have inspired me to be even better in all aspects of life.

Ankit

Acknowledgements

From Julie

There are so many people in my little universe to whom I am grateful—and that universe expanded tremendously when I added Breast Cancer Survivor to my life experience resumé. I can't begin to acknowledge them all.... but I can try!

To my family who continue to support and tolerate and help me to have enough time to write "on the side". You are the light of my life.

To my amazing staff at Pediatric Partners of Ponte Vedra without whom I would not get through one day. My gratitude knows no bounds.

To Janeen Herskovitz, Amy Groshell, Marie Walchle and the phenomenal support team that propped up my family and me. You made sure we were fed and errands were run, and you marshaled what has to have been the largest, most powerful, most amazing, most intensely prayerful group of people who have ever gathered for one purpose across this big wide world. Thank God for email, and thank God for each of you. Ours was the very most amazing 14-hour Angel Party I will ever have the good fortune to attend!

To Peggy Neville, my breast care coordinator. When you looked straight into my eyes, I saw an angel. When I told you I was writing a book about integrative care for breast cancer patients, you said, "I'm so sorry for you, but I'm so glad for all of the women who always want to know how to do the integrative part. Now they'll have a resource." Here it is, Peggles.

To Mary Alderman, the first doctor I had had in more than five years, and to Ankit Desai, Unni Thomas and Gary Bowers, the treating team that she assembled when I would have no part of it. Thank you thank you thank you for helping me stumble, as gracefully as possible, through a process that was never a part of my life plan. The outcome has been absolutely amazing!

To Stephanie Cave, my friend, and my integrative genius guru. I'll never forget calling you to say I couldn't come and visit right now because I had been diagnosed with breast cancer. Your response was, "Do you have a pencil? Start writing." This book includes all of the words I wrote that day. Big hugs and lots of gratitude.

To Joan Ryan, Michele Palumbo, Bill Schindler, Samir Patel, and the rest of the folks who contributed to and comprised my Integrative Approach Team. You have truly made all of the difference as I walk the road less travelled.

To Karen and Frank Brower and the entire Brower clan. The respite and glorious solitude of your "cabin" in Maine was a writing haven. The blessing of meals shared with a very big "family" for a long weekend were the stuff of which lasting and loving memories are made. Thank you.

To Lynn Vannucci who has an amazing talent for getting the thoughts in my head into some sort of readable organization. I love how it comes together!

Publishing in the new digital model is different in so many ways from traditional publishing—thank you to the entire crew at Water Street Press for a wonderful experience. Who knew that there were so many jobs and processes to get a book from our heads into readers' hands!

From Ankit

This will never be all encompassing, but let me try:

To my wife, Mittal, and daughter, Karina, for their love and support and for all the happiness they bring into my life.

To my parents, Mala & Rajni, who provided me with more than any son could ask for.

To my family Niral, Alpesh, Tarak, Indravadan, & Saudamini for all that they do.

To my office family and partner, Michael Fallucco, who share with me my passion for plastic surgery and allow me to perform my profession with such joy and ease.

To Lynn Vannucci, for all of her wondrous ability and motivation to make this book become a reality.

And to Julie Buckley for being an inspiration, and for making me a part of her journey and this book. She is no longer only my patient, but also a lifelong friend.

About the Authors

Julie A. Buckley, MD is the author of *Healing Our Autistic Children: A Medical Plan for Restoring Your Child's Health*. She practices functional medicine in Ponte Vedra Beach, Florida (www.pppvonline.com) where she lives with her husband and two children.

Dr. Ankit Desai is a board certified cosmetic and reconstructive plastic surgeon practicing in Jacksonville, Florida (www.plasticsurgeryjacksonville.com) where he lives with his wife and daughter.

Contents

Foreword

Spotlight on Breast Cancer

I think of myself as a small town girl, happiest at home, surrounded by my family. I've never sought the spotlight, and I surely am not comfortable in it. But when you're married to Brett Favre, a famous NFL quarterback, the spotlight is always on him and it's hard to avoid. As his wife, I have worked hard to be graceful in that spotlight.

With our blessings come, we feel, a certain responsibility. Since 1995, Brett and I have worked to help disadvantaged and differently abled kids through the Make a Wish Foundation, Special Olympics, and the Association for Rights of Mentally Handicapped Citizens. Part of the 'good' of doing this work has been, of course, that we have been a part of helping to heal and improve the lives of these kids—the smiles and the high fives we've received from the kids themselves have warmed our hearts and brought us joy.

Another part of the 'good' is the way this work has helped to heal and improve *our* lives. Brett and I have faced challenges just like any other couple—we've dealt with hardship and stress. But, amazingly, by doing almost instinctively what my friend Pastor Shane Stanford and I articulated in our book, *The Cure for the Chronic Life*—reaching outward in the hope of bringing comfort to others—we reaped comfort for ourselves.

Then, in 2004, I was diagnosed with breast cancer. You're reading a book called *Breast Cancer: Start Here*, so my guess is you know how this diagnosis rocks your world—ushers in the incredible hardship of sickness and vulnerability of stress. As Julie and Ankit explain in this book, the average breast cancer patient has about a month between the day she is diagnosed and the day she begins treatment. A month to battle through an onslaught of emotions, to be sad, inconvenienced, scared and angry and work her way toward resolute, and determined, all while learning and reading and preparing and interviewing doctors and weighing one treatment option against seven others and informing friends and helping family and oneself to get ready for a big journey into the unknown.

A diagnosis of breast cancer, while it is the most personal of events, is actually one that forces you to handle it fairly publicly. It may be a time when we want to wallow in denial and anger, but in order to survive we can't focus for long on our negative feelings. We must take positive action, seek advice and help and knowledge. We must turn outward in the most intimate ways.

I wish this book had been available to me when I was first beginning my breast cancer journey. The choices I made nine years ago might have been different in terms of the treatments available at the time and those available now, certainly; but what would have made a world of difference is having this comprehensive yet concise, straightforward yet optimistic, no-nonsense yet funny and loving book to guide me on my path to survivorship.

And I am a survivor. I am one of that select 'Steel Magnolia' sorority Julie describes. After my recovery, Brett and I expanded the scope of our foundation's portfolio—the spotlight I have had to embrace has allowed me the opportunity to raise awareness about the disease I have beaten, and to raise funds in support of women who were not, as I was, lucky enough to have the resources to fight the disease. As a survivor, I transitioned from breast cancer patient to breast cancer advocate. I'm thankful to have another opportunity to reach outward today—to shine the spotlight on a book that I believe can help to heal and improve and *save* the lives of women who, like me, have been diagnosed with breast cancer.

Deanna Favre
Favre4Hope Foundation
www.favre4hope.com
November 2013

Introduction

Physician, Healing Myself

What I had needed was a guide to help me understand and maintain breast health. What I needed now, right away, immediately, was a way to navigate the traditional options for breast cancer treatment—mastectomy and chemo and reconstruction—that also helped me understand how non-traditional therapies could boost my odds of beating this disease. What I was going to need was a handbook that outlined the things I could do to keep my breast cancer from recurring—because, make no mistake, I was going to beat cancer. Anything else was not an option. But the book I needed did not exist. 'OK, Julie,' I told myself, 'there's your next project. Go write that book.'

Julie Buckley, MD

In July 2009, as my book, *Healing Our Autistic Children*, was being readied for publication, I was diagnosed with breast cancer. My first thought as my doctor gave me this news is unprintable—I was a sailor before I attended medical school. After that, my responses were a jumble. Being a doctor myself, specializing in cutting-edge biomedical treatment of autism spectrum diseases, I am trained to be—when I have to be—the bearer of similarly hard news; surely, even as the recipient of this "you have cancer" bombshell, some part of me remained professionally detached, alert to the medical information at hand and ready to chart a course for treatment. I'm an optimist by nature so, certainly, it must have crossed my mind that whatever treatment options lay before me I was going to give this cancer one hell of a run for its money. I love life—for all of its challenges, I love *my* life—so don't doubt for a moment that this abrupt, complicated confrontation with mortality filled me with grief.

But the first rational, fully formed thoughts I remember having, a split second after the gravity of my doctor's words threatened to blow my mind, were, *How am I going to tell my children I have cancer? Who's going to take care of my family while I'm in treatment? What are my patients going to do while I'm out of commission? Doctors don't get sick!*

And then I laughed. Out loud. Which startled my doctor and forced me to explain myself.

For years I had been preaching to the parents of my young autism patients about the importance of taking care of themselves—*taking care of the caretaker*. Being a caretaker, I reminded them at every opportunity, is demanding, stressful work. It is critical that Mom and Dad—and Grandpa and Grandma, brother and sister, aunt and uncle and godparent and whoever else is part of any sick child's primary support team—keep up their own health in order to provide the child with quality care. When I gave these "take care of yourself" sermons to my patients' parents, however, I wasn't talking only about remaining physically fit so that they would be able to dispense medicines, change diapers, and drive their children to therapy appointments. In fact, I was speaking primarily of emotional health—of maintaining a home environment that was as calm and low-stress as possible because *serenity is central to healing*. I was able to speak these words with a great deal of credibility: I am not only a doctor; I am also the mother of an autistic child. I have first-hand experience of how severe the costs of neglecting a caretaker's psychological well-being can be. For instance, the accumulated emotional stress of caregiving can play havoc with relationships. Eighty percent of autistic children grow up in homes that become single-parent households after the child's diagnosis, because of the stress of raising a child with special needs can be so overwhelming. Thankfully, my strong and intact family was testimony to our coping skills.

But stress is a many-tentacled monster. It not only hampers the healing of the sick and wrecks relationships; stress is also a huge factor in the *development* of real, physical disease. The weight of simple, everyday stress can lead to illness for the caretaker him- or herself. *Serenity is central to not getting sick in the first place.* This statement is not just some new-age sound bite trying to pass itself off as fact. The science has been accumulating for over a decade.

Stress—strain, anxiety, worry, nervous tension—is not merely an emotional condition. It is the word we use to describe authentic physical circumstances: clenched teeth, knotted muscles, rising blood pressure, aching head, roiling tummy, insomnia.

At the most basic level, we can say that stress is the response humans have to the external factors of our lives—our jobs, our relationships, the environments we live in. It is our reactions to the difficulties and challenges we face on a daily basis, and these reactions are shaped in large part by the expectations we have in any particular situation. Did we *expect* a project to proceed smoothly? Did we *expect* to get that promotion after putting in two weeks of all-nighters on that project at work, or did we *expect* to finish giving the kitchen a new coat of paint over the weekend? The natural stresses of everyday living are exacerbated when our expectations are not met—when the promotion falls through, or the dog barrels through the backdoor upsetting the gallon of paint and making it necessary for us to spend the first four hours of project time scrubbing robin's egg blue paint out of the white grouting on our tile floor.

How we handle the aggravated stress imposed on us by *external* factors, however, varies from person to person, depending in great part on *internal* factors. Do we eat a wholesome, nutritionally balanced diet? Do we get enough sleep? Do we exercise and stay fit? Do we enjoy overall health? Are our relationships generally satisfactory and emotionally secure? Folks who can answer "yes" to these simple but telling questions are likely able to respond to stress in more productive and proactive ways than those who subsist on fast food meals, lead sedentary lifestyles, or have tumultuous primary relationships. The headaches, muscles aches and tension, digestion issues, sleep problems and fatigue that are associated with stress are often much less severe when our general physical and emotional equilibrium is in good order.

This is not to say that all stress is bad. The "fight or flight response" we experience when we are confronted with a situation that we perceive as dangerous, for example, is a form of stress that is—in small, quick, *acute* doses—beneficial. When we see a large, unleashed, barking dog along our path or a driver overshoots a stop sign and is suddenly in our lane, our adrenal gland reacts by releasing *neurotransmitters*. Neurotransmitters are the chemicals our body produces that allow our nerves to talk to each other. In case of danger, the two neurotransmitters that are released are epinephrine (more commonly called adrenaline) and norepinephrine. These neurotransmitters cause physical responses—an increased heart rate and a heightened sense of alertness that works to our advantage in dealing with a strange, angry dog or swerving to avoid a collision. Stress has a purpose.

But when there is an overabundance of it in lives, or when we cope with it in unhealthy ways—from "merely" not permitting ourselves the time and peace to recover from our daily doses of it to the extremes of overeating or using alcohol, tobacco, or harder drugs—we set up a chain reaction in our bodies that is far more dangerous than your average unleashed barking dog. The accumulation of daily stress causes *oxidative stress* and a *chronic inflammatory response*. And cumulative chronic oxidative stress and inflammatory responses can be both the cause of and evidence of a body starting to break down; they are what pave the dark way toward grave and life-threatening diseases like breast cancer.

Let's be clear about this at the outset: disease is a path, or a *process*. That process may be longer or shorter for different people, and the way that disease manifests may be different as well—breast cancer, heart disease, autism, Alzheimer's—depending on a myriad of environmental, lifestyle and genetic variables. How directly and quickly we walk the path toward disease, however, is quite often within our control. We all know that smoking cigarettes, for instance, is a path to lung cancer, emphysema, heart disease and other circulatory diseases. This is science that is no longer disputed by even the most aggressive tobacco interests: cigarettes are a straight and frequently fast sprint toward illness. By quitting smoking, or by never even starting to smoke, we reduce the chance that we may end up on the lung cancer path.

What many of us may not yet be familiar with are the subtle, *specific* ways in which cigarettes cause disease—or the ways in which less obvious assaults on the body can cause the same subtle physiological effects that can, cumulatively, lead to diseases just as devastating.

Oxidative Stress. We are all familiar with what can happen to our cars when we leave them exposed to too much rain and wind and sun without a good coat of wax to protect them. They rust. Chemists call this *oxidation* and what they mean by that is the process by which electrons are removed from atoms and molecules by interaction with too much oxygen, causing corrosion. In our bodies, the same sort of "corrosion" can take place. How does this happen? In order to create the energy we need to work and play and live our daily lives, we eat food. The digested food is turned into fuel when it is *metabolized*—that is, when it is combined with the air that we breathe, specifically through a metabolic process called *catabolism*. Unfortunately, this process of creating fuel also creates unwanted—and dangerous—byproducts, called *free radicals*.

Free radicals are electronically unstable atoms. This means that they don't have all the electrons they need to be complete. In order to complete themselves they run frantically amok, stealing electrons from other, stable atoms in the body and—as a result—leaving ever more unstable atoms in their wake. Free radicals, in essence, break down the very structure of our cells; so much so that the cells are vulnerable and unable to do their part in supporting life. The purpose of many of our cells is to repair our genetic structure as we continue to age and to prevent unwanted changes that can result in disease. The destruction of these cells has been implicated in diseases from autism to atherosclerosis to rapid aging, Parkinson's to Alzheimer's, heart failure to—yes—cancer.

Further, free radicals are created not only through the catabolic process. They are also the result of environmental pressures such as toxins in food (think of the petrochemical fertilizers that have, since the 1950s, become common in agribusiness to grow our fruits and vegetables), in water (think of the mercury released into the air from your area's coal-fired power plant; the mercury lands on the ground and is eventually flushed into rivers and reservoirs for you to drink—and to be eaten by the fish that you, in turn, consume), and in the air (think of the exhaust fumes from cars and trucks and belching buses). Now, think even harder—there are harmful toxins that put pressure on our human biological systems in nearly every mundane thing we touch nearly every day: the aluminum in many deodorants, the BPAs in our plastic water bottles, the amalgams in our dental fillings, the chemicals in cleaning products and pest control sprays and hair dyes and the chemical make up of many brands of cosmetics. While over the last ten or twenty years it has become much more widely known within the general population that the chemicals in everyday products are harmful to us in a myriad of terrible ways—a quick, random Google search netted this article about birth defects that have been linked to glyphosate, the "chemical at the heart of the planet's most widely used herbicide, Roundup weedkiller"[1]—regulation of such dangerous substances remains elusive; it is nearly impossible to avoid coming into contact with some sort of environmental stress factor in the course of modern life.

This constant bombardment of toxins is one of the reasons that it's important to take daily vitamin supplements with good doses of Vitamins C and E. These vitamins in particular can counter some of the effects of oxidative stress because they are "donors"—literally offering some of their electrons to the free radicals and stabilizing them, repairing some of the damage that toxins have caused and often preventing cellular "suicide", an act our cells are programmed to perform if they are too damaged to recover. Often, unfortunately, these supplements alone are not enough to combat and win both emotional and environmental stress assaults.

---

1 http://www.huffingtonpost.com/2011/06/24/roundup-scientists-birth-defects_n_883578.html.

Chronic Inflammatory Response. When we bang our shins against a table, slice a finger instead of the apple we were paring, or are exposed to a flu virus, our bodies respond with one of their most basic protective functions: inflammatory response. This response sends cells and biochemicals to the site of the bruise, the cut, the cluster of foreign virus particles to do battle and begin the healing process. We can see, and often feel, the body's attempt to heal itself—redness, a localized warmth, swelling, even tiredness, bleeding and pain can be clues that our body's defenses have kicked in and are addressing the injury we have sustained or the disease that has invaded our system. This rush to defense is an *acute inflammatory response*; it is immediate, beneficial, and short-lived.

Chronic inflammatory response, however, is what happens when the body's urge to repair itself goes into overdrive *because the insult it has sustained is, or is perceived to be, continuous.* Here is a most amazing biological fact: the body won't stop trying to repair itself just because it hasn't yet been successful at the task. Its defense operations are diligent, and tenacious, but fairly easily confused: when the inflammatory response is prolonged the cells and biochemicals the body dispatches to tend to the insult can start to attack healthy cells and tissues, simultaneously healing and causing more damage.

Let's say, for example, that you have gone out to lunch and, in the course of the meal, spilled coffee on your favorite white shirt. You didn't notice the spill at first and, by the time you get home, the stain has pretty much set. You pull out a clean cloth and some solvent and begin to work on the stain and, at first, the stain begins to fade so you think your efforts to save the shirt are paying off. The stain is stubborn, however, so you pour a little more solvent on it, rub a little harder. Eventually you may succeed at removing the stain, but at the cost of having treated the fabric so harshly that you've damaged the fibers, weakening their strength, changing their texture or color, or even making a hole in the garment.

In the body, the long-term effects of chronic inflammation are similar: the cells and tissues are weakened, their structures altered, and holes, or wounds, begin to appear in the tissue. And, when cells and tissues are compromised in this manner, we are more vulnerable to disease. Chronic inflammation has been linked to a diverse array of disorders—asthma and Alzheimer's, cirrhosis of the liver, psoriasis, chronic bowel disease, heartburn, the painful muscle disorder known as fibromyalgia, diabetes, meningitis and cystic fibrosis. And even cancer.[2]

Take, for example, the bacteria known as Helicobacter pylori, or H. pylori. It is estimated that nearly half of the world's population is currently infected with H. pylori, which grows only in the stomach, weakening its protective coating so that digestive juices begin to irritate the delicate stomach lining.[3] It is responsible for most ulcers and many cases of stom-

---

2 http://www.cdc.gov/ncidod/eid/vol4no3/cassell.htm.

3 http://www.ncbi.nlm.nih.gov/pubmedhealth/PMH0001276/.

ach inflammation, or what is also called chronic gastritis.[4] A 1994 study by the International Agency for Research on Cancer concluded that human H. pylori infection is associated with the risk of developing adenocarcinoma (i.e., cancer) of the stomach, one of the most common malignancies in the world, as well as two other types of cancers.[5]

Think of it: one of every two people in the world is infected with cancer-causing stomach bacteria. No wonder chronic inflammation is such a silent epidemic. An alarming statistic is that over 50% of American adults and children are currently on some form of medication for chronic illness.[6] This includes almost two-thirds of women over twenty years of age, over half of adult men, one in four children and teens, and three in four adults over sixty-five.[7]

Chronic inflammatory response and oxidative stress are both contributors to and evidence of disease processes in our bodies—this, science knows for sure.

What it also knows for sure is that chronic inflammatory response and oxidative stress are part of the *aging process*. Now, I don't want to get in trouble—I don't want any of you to think

---

4 Ibid.

5 http://www.cdc.gov/ncidod/eid/vol4no3/cassell.htm.

6 http://www.foxnews.com/story/0,2933,355540,00.html.

7 Ibid.

that I regard aging as a disease; quite the contrary, aging is a privilege. It is, as any cancer survivor will tell you, also a real, true joy. But as we age, our bodies—our cells—begin to feel the cumulative effects of a lifetime of various stresses; they become more fragile and less able to cope with the assaults of everyday stress. Here, however, is the disturbing part of how—and how fast—a cell loses its ability to cope with stress in our modern world: When I was a child, chronic inflammation and oxidative stress caught up to my friends' grandparents when they were in their seventies and they'd end up having to take daily medication for some sort of illness. Then it was our grandparents in their sixties losing their health. Next thing I knew it was people who were in their fifties having to pick up monthly meds at the pharmacy. And then it was me, in my forties. What has happened to us as a population, as a culture, that we are getting—and staying—sick at younger and younger ages? Quite simply, the toxic physical environment we have created for ourselves to live in has increased our experience of oxidative stress and chronic inflammatory response to dangerous levels—from the chemicals that are used to grow our foods and the heavy metals that are the by-products of fossil fuel consumption, to the everyday pace of modern life that can be *emotionally* toxic. The recuperative abilities of our bodies, their innate repair and restore responses, have been exceeded by the demands we are placing upon them with these excessive myriad environmental exposures.

༈

There are only four kinds of people

in the world—those who have been

caretakers, those who are currently

caretakers, those who will be caretakers,

and those who will need care.

Former First Lady, Rosalyn Carter

For caretakers, however, there is yet another wrinkle in the disease process—and this extra wrinkle should truly be a global concern because every single one of us is or will be a caretaker at some point in our lives. Parents and teachers, therapists and health care professionals like myself, Baby Boomers who are responsible for the care of aging parents, the spouses of people who suffer from debilitating diseases or injury—few of us will get through life without some greater or lesser period of stress created by a loved one's sickness, and that means pretty much all of us face an additional risk factor.

So here's the bad news. In 2006, researchers at the Department of General Internal Medicine at University Hospital in Switzerland found stunning biochemical evidence of the impact of stress on caretakers.[8] Biochemistry is, simply, the

---

8 http://www.ncbi.nlm.nih.gov/pubmed/16960028.

study of the natural, biologically occurring chemical compounds that sustain life. In this instance, the compound the researchers were studying was Interleukin-6, a protein that, in the human body, is encoded by the IL-6 gene. IL-6 is one of the most well studied human genes because it plays such a significant role in our health. It is one of the most important mediators of the body's response to fevers and other acute inflammations. But, as with almost anything else, moderation is the key with IL-6. Just as drinking one glass of red wine with dinner might be helpful in preventing heart disease but drinking a bottle of wine every night can be a factor in the cause of disease, when a body overproduces IL-6, problems result. In the most benign cases, these problems manifest as higher rates of infection, colds, and influenza. But the problems associated with an oversupply of IL-6 can also be far more grave, including higher incidence of diseases such as diabetes, atherosclerosis, and cancer, to name a few. When researchers discovered that elevated levels of IL-6 were routinely found in the blood of advanced, or metastatic, cancer patients, they began to develop anti-IL-6 agents to combat disease. The first successful anti-IL-6 agent is called tocilizumab, which has been approved for use in treating rheumatoid arthritis; other anti-IL-6 agents are, as I write, in clinical trials.

What is most pertinent to our immediate discussion, however, is the link that researchers at Ohio State were able to make between IL-6 and caregiving. They discovered that the stress of caregiving in the population they studied caused the production of IL-6 to increase *four times faster* than the normal rate.⁹ The people who are responsible for the care of a sick loved one—such as the parents of my young patients—are at real risk for a variety of life-threatening illnesses.

But, as we've already noted, it isn't only the parents of autistic children who are caregivers, of course. And the 2003 Ohio State study wasn't the only one to indicate that caregivers are at risk. Also in 2003, for example, a study conducted by the Harvard School of Public Health[10] found that for women caregivers—and, let's face it, women are the world's primary caregivers—the downsides of caregiving included the risk of increased incidence of coronary heart disease; the Harvard study sheds a harsh light on one of the reasons why women suffer disproportionately from heart disease: it is the number one killer of women in the United States today.[11]

Way back in 1999, a study by the Department of Psychiatry and University Center for Social and Urban Research at the University of Pittsburgh focused on older caregivers. Their premise was that "the combination of loss, prolonged distress, the physical demands of caregiving, and biological vulnerability of older caregivers may compromise their physiological functioning and increase their risk for physical health problems."[12] Their conclusion, sadly, validated their theory. The researchers found that older caregivers were, indeed, more

---

9 http://www.ncbi.nlm.nih.gov/pubmed/12840146.

10 http://www.ajpmonline.org/article/S0749-3797(02)00582-2/abstract.

11 http://www.nlm.nih.gov/medlineplus/heartdiseaseinwomen.html.

12 http://www.ucsur.pitt.edu/files/schulz/AJGPEditorial.pdf.

likely to die from the strain associated with caregiving than their non-caregiving counterparts.[13]

I had long known about such studies. They were among the reasons I'd always been so adamant that my patients' parents eat well and take appropriate dietary supplements; go into the hyperbaric chamber with their child every chance they got; make time for date nights with their partner. *Tend to yourselves*, I pleaded with them. I had even gone so far as to counsel my professional peers—teachers, therapists, and other doctors who work in the high-stress world of healing—to be mindful of their own vulnerability. So the irony was not lost on me as I sat in my doctor's office with my new diagnosis of cancer. I was the physician who had not cared for herself, the cobbler whose children had no shoes. In spite of what I had long known intellectually, I had not *acted on* my knowledge—beyond an hour stolen here and there to take a yoga class, what had I been doing to take care of *me*? Like most of the parents I preached to, I rarely found the time to indulge myself. Pampering Dr. Julie with the little luxuries—a massage, a romantic dinner with my husband, a shopping spree at my local bookstore to stock up on pleasure reading—were often beyond the family budget. Asking for the help that might have provided me with the time to actually sit down in a cozy chair and indulge in an hour of pleasure reading did not—as I suspect it does not for many caregivers—come easily to me.

---

13 http://jama.ama-assn.org/content/282/23/2215.full.

Even as I chastised myself for neglecting my own health, however, I knew with guilty certainty that the little time for yoga that I did manage to sneak into my schedule was likely a whole lot more than most caregivers were able to give themselves. This grim reality—this lack of wherewithal, be it the time or the energy or the money necessary to make oneself a priority from time to time—was the basis for a crisis in the making.

At this point, I think it is worth taking the notion of what creates stress just one step further. It is not only someone else's medical upheavals that drain us of physical, mental and emotional energy. How many times have you used the word "stress" to explain the result of trying to balance the demands of home life with the demands of a full-time job? To describe the feeling of waiting on hold for the technician to tell you how to fix your computer; the minutes ticking by, the deadline for that report your boss needs on her desk that very afternoon growing ever more slender? The feeling of utter frustration when you take your car in for routine service and find out that having the oil changed is the smallest—and the least expensive— of the old heap's problems? The feeling of breathlessness in the morning when you look at your day's schedule and realize that your daughter has an appointment with the dentist and a dance lesson after school, your son has a basketball game and a Cub Scout meeting in the evening, it's time to give the dog his monthly dose of heartworm medication and you're out of pills, your spouse is out of town on a business trip and you have promised the PTA that you will bring a batch of cookies by to contribute to their bake sale. A hypothetical, nearly comical array of issues, you say? We have one friend, a single mom who is raising three teenagers, teaching full-time in an autistic classroom, and taking credits toward her master's degree—and we were not surprised when she was recently diagnosed with Graves' Disease.[14] Caretaking our own daily lives is stressful. We are all at risk.

Well, now I was the one who was sick. My own daily stress of balancing a home life and a career—caring for my autistic daughter, my teenage son, my husband and home; maintaining medical practices in two different cities and flying all over the world to present at medical conferences and mentor other doctors—had manifested itself as breast cancer. Now I had no choice but to slow down and "indulge" myself. Take time off. Ask for help. I had *cancer*. I had to become my own priority. Honestly, at first blush, the mere thought of that exhausted me; I was just one more thing to add to my already unwieldy to-do list.

It's fortunate that my husband and I have a long-standing arrangement for what happens in our house when one or the other of us has come to the end of our physical energy or emotional inspiration. The one of us who is exhausted will simply

---

14 The most common form of hyperthyroidism that occurs when the body's immune system mistakenly attacks the thyroid gland, causing it to overproduce the hormone thyroxine.

say to the other, "You're lead dog tonight," and the designated alpha dog never questions the reason. The lead dog gets to gather the family for dinner, wash the dishes, supervise homework, make sure the kids have baths and get to bed on time, and mediate any common family crisis that comes up while the house is running on his or her watch. The phone rings? The lead dog answers it. The kids can't agree on a video to watch? Lead dog's problem. Football practice starts the next day? Lead dog signs the consent form and makes sure we can locate the shoulder pads and washes the uniform so it's ready to go in the morning.

The night after I was diagnosed with cancer, lead dog was a role that both my husband and I recognized was going to be his for a good many months ahead, and he stepped right into it without my having to even ask. All I wanted was a hot bath. I needed a long soak in some steaming water to clear my head before we told the kids that I was sick. Before I told my mother and enlisted even extra helpings of her already generously given time. Before I could figure out what in the world to tell my patients.

I had every intention of getting into the tub to meditate but conscious thought persisted. *Well. Cancer. This is just terribly inconvenient.* We were in the middle of training Flux, my daughter's new autism service dog; would I have the energy for a new puppy in the house? I was scheduled to speak at two national conferences, to present new research on hyperbarics to my peers; would I be able to travel during chemo? My book was being released in six months and there would be speaking engagements and book signings associated with that event; I couldn't be bald! In addition to being an autism specialist, I am the personal physician to several NFL players and these young men, their wives and girlfriends and children have become part of our extended family—like extra sons and daughters to my husband and me; one of my players had recently been traded and I had plans in place to take my children across the country for a long weekend to see him play for his new team. How was I supposed to work *that* around my chemo schedule?

These thoughts and more were crowding for room inside my brain. Untangling them and shutting them up seemed overwhelming so I decided, since I couldn't find that quiet space I craved inside my own head, I might as well do something useful while I was up to my neck in hot water. I started to wash myself. When I got to my feet I lingered for a few seconds, massaging the area at the top of my foot, just below my toes. As I did this I felt a tremendous surge of well being and, before I could consciously wonder why, I realized that I was paying attention to the part of the foot that reflexologists associate with breast health. Nearly instantly I felt calmer, better, just by doing one thing that took almost no time, and cost nothing. And I began to feel a tingling—the delightful excitement of discovery.

As I dried off and climbed into my pajamas, the feeling grew. What are the things that caregivers can do to protect their health, or to get their health back on track if, like me, their train had been derailed? What diet item or items were most important? What vitamin supplement? What therapy—

massage, hyperbarics, anti-oxidant infusions—would give already overworked and budget-conscious caretakers the most bang for their buck?

The various studies that had been—and are being—conducted around the world that focus on the risks associated with caregiver health were clear evidence that I wasn't the only caregiver who was going down for the count. In fact, the epidemic of illness we are facing today—sharp rises in the rates of autism[15], cancer[16], Alzheimer's[17], just for a few examples—indicates a correlating epidemic of caregiver distress and disease to come. Perhaps if I could explain why caregivers were so stressed—the biochemistry of stress and how it can lead to disease—caregivers would take their own health, and the measures they can employ to preserve it, more seriously. I had learned the hard way what could happen to my ability to serve those who depended on me when I didn't pay attention to my own health. But I was also a doctor who had immersed herself for years in the biomedical, functional medicine model for healing disease and relieving pain—how could I apply the tools that were already in my toolbox to my own needs? Perhaps if, as I went through cancer treatment employing the tools that were at my disposal, I could offer my experience, and the knowledge I gained from it, as an example of how to

---

15 http://www.nlm.nih.gov/medlineplus/news/fullstory_112355.html.

16 http://www.who.int/mediacentre/news/releases/2003/pr27/en/.

17 http://www.sciencedaily.com/releases/2007/06/070610104441.htm.

integrate these tools into other caregivers' tight schedules, and likely even tighter budgets.

My immediate concern, of course, was cancer. My own illness. How could I deploy the tools that were already in my toolbox to fighting breast cancer? What treatments would boost the efficacy of the more traditional, cancer-specific treatments I now faced? How would hyperbarics, antioxidant infusions, supplements and diet and the like enhance what the general surgeon and medical oncologist were already planning to do for me? And, not incidentally, how would they help me through whatever process of breast reconstruction I was going to choose? What was the science behind how these non-traditional treatments would work? As I had done when my daughter, Dani, was diagnosed with autism, I would have to go back and do yet another residency—this time not about the biomedical approach to autism, but about the biomedical approach to disease prevention and healing for breast cancer patients, like myself. If I could produce a concise and accessible collection of the best of this emerging new science, perhaps then other women wouldn't have to learn the hard way.

What I had needed was a guide to help me understand and maintain breast health. But what I needed now, right away, immediately, was a way to navigate the traditional options for breast cancer treatment—mastectomy and chemo and reconstruction—that also helped me understand how non-traditional therapies could boost my odds of beating this disease. What I was going to need was a handbook that outlined the things I could do to keep my breast cancer from recurring—

because, make no mistake, I was going to beat cancer. Anything else was not an option. But the book I needed did not exist. *OK, Julie*, I told myself, *there's your next project. Go write that book.*

To do this, I knew I was going to have to find a partner. Someone who knew more about breast cancer and breast reconstruction and *breasts* than I did. I did not know at the time that this person was going to be my brilliant breast reconstruction surgeon, Ankit Desai. At that point Ankit and I hadn't yet even met—and I had not yet conceived what would become my first and most basic rule for women who are diagnosed with breast cancer: however counterintuitive this advice might sound the first time you hear it, I think it is critical that, before a breast cancer patient chooses her general surgeon and oncologist, she must choose her reconstructive surgeon. As I buttoned my pajamas and slipped into my fuzzy slippers that first night that I was diagnosed, however, I had faith that this person, my partner, would appear in the course of my treatment.

I am a firm believer that "things" happen for a reason. Breast cancer was my opportunity to slow down, to give myself a time-out from the everyday stressors of life and focus my energy on *me*. To have permission to pour love on myself as much as I poured love on everyone else. To catch up on all the sleep I'd missed over the years to be with my kids, and my husband, and my patients. To change my life forever—radically and all at once—for the better; to walk the walk rather than just talk the talk about the healthy, lower stress lifestyle

I advised for everyone else. To take off the roller blades and put out the fire that always seemed to be at my back, driving me forward, and to tend to my own free radicals and chronic aches and pains, get my own biochemistry balanced. Breast cancer, viewed from this perspective, was a gift. Surely if God was going to give me such a big gift, He was also going to send me the person I needed in order to figure out how to unwrap it and put it to its best use!

I brushed my hair and tied it back in a ponytail. I sighed then, knowing that I wasn't going to have much longer to worry about what to do with my hair. But it was a brief moment of sadness. Yes, I was going to lose my hair; but it would eventually, of course, grow back. Meantime, I was now fully located in the calm, quiet place I'd been trying to force myself to reach when I'd first walked into the bathroom to soak. I'd found a purpose to my illness, and a practical way to deal with it. I knew that first thing in the morning I was going to call my editor and start to talk with her about my next book—sharing the tools of health, the why and how of adapting and applying them to breast cancer recovery and breast health. That night I had a genuine smile on my face as I tied my robe around my waist, opened the bathroom door and called to my husband so we could go out to the living room together and tell the kids that I was sick.

Julie Buckley, MD
August 2013

1

What is Breast Cancer?

No wonder we're confused about breasts.

Julie

Is there any other part of the human

body that has been as celebrated, as censored, and as subject to the whim of fashion as the female breast?

Earliest man, way back two or three million years ago in the Stone Age, lacking any concepts of agriculture or the alphabet and all but the most rudimentary flaked-stone tools, knew one thing with absolute certainty: the female breast was awfully handy for feeding the babies. It was the only thing that stood between the survival of their tribes and extinction by attrition. This is why we see big-breasted, and even many-breasted stone, clay, and bone figurines among the most notable artifacts of the age: breasts represented abundance, the very font of life, and so, for ancient man, they were elevated to the sacred.

Later, the Greeks, a more "sophisticated"[18] bunch, narrowed the object of worship from two breasts to one phallus, and breasts were not only demoted but became suspect: the

---

18 From the Greek *sophistikos*, which means of or pertaining to a sophist: a wise man.

Greeks invented the legend of the Amazon,[19] warrior women who chopped off one breast in order to more efficiently draw their dangerous bows, though they left the other breast intact in order to nurse their female children—because, of course, these powerful if mythical women disposed of any male offspring.

In the Dark Ages, the Roman Catholic Church was not well disposed toward the human body in general and the art of the time reflects this—it is nearly impossible to tell the girls from the boys—though in the Renaissance, emphasis once again returned to the flesh and the female breast, in count-less paintings of Madonna and Child, became the symbol of maternal love as well as spiritual nourishment. In the 15th cen-tury the image of the breast once again took a turn for the worse: paintings often depicted couples with the husband's hand cupping the wife's breast, as a way to demonstrate his ownership; in the 18th century the "domestic breast" got a lot of attention as the medical community decided it didn't like the practice of wet-nursing and that even wealthy women should nurse their own children. The 19th century saw a fash-ion for full bosoms—and the invention of a suction device, painful to even contemplate, designed to increase the bust size of the less naturally endowed; in the 20th century, women in the 1960s burned their bras as a way of proving they could, at

---

19 From the Greek *a*, meaning "without", and *mazos*, meaning "breast".

last, do what they wanted with their own ta-tas, perhaps as a counter to a cultural obsession summed up some years later by humorist Dave Barry: "Scientists now believe that the primary biological function of breasts is to make men stupid."

The beautiful, functional breast has spent centuries as the focus of religious censorship, political statements, fashion trends and lust, this latter frequently of the anonymous sort. Faced with cancer and the potential imminent loss of my own, it struck me what an odd, onerous burden breasts have historically had to bear. Couldn't one simply *like* one's own breasts? Simply because they *were* beautiful and functional? My breasts had been part of my life for nearly thirty years, old friends— *the girls*—and I grieved for them. I remember lying on my doctor's examination table, looking at a poster of flowers stuck to the examining room wall, and shedding some hot tears while I waited for yet another pre-op medical procedure. My grief, however, was, as I imagine it is for many women who face the same diagnosis, very *personal*. I didn't think of my breasts as flagships of womanhood or motherhood; I thought that they had given *me* so much pleasure; they had fed *my* children. Now they had, in all likelihood, to go, and saying goodbye was going to be hard.

Let me hasten to add at this point that I never gave the cancer surgery a second thought. Having the mastectomies was an absolute no-brainer for me. Maybe it was because I am blessed with such a solid marriage, and my husband didn't give the surgery a second thought himself. Maybe it was because I had already been through so many medical trials— back surgery that was supposed to have permanently disabled me and did not; raising an autistic child—that cancer seemed like just another thing that I'd have to deal with. Maybe it was because my mother is a thirty-year breast cancer survivor, so I had living proof that surgery was the right thing to do. Or maybe it was because I'd watched my father's Hodgkin's lymphoma progress over the course of my young life, and saw the lengths to which he went in order to be around a few years longer, and then a few months longer, a struggle he waged primarily so that he could be there for me as I grew up. "The alternative," he once told me, "is just unacceptable." I knew I had to do what I had to do in order to watch my own kids grow up. It was that simple.

So, before the doctor came in to do the procedure I was waiting for, I had a heart-to-heart talk with my breasts. "Thank you," I told them. "Thank you for nurturing my children. Thank you for all the fun you've given me. But now you've got something going on inside you that I don't want in my body, and it's time to swap you out for a new pair…"

Having breast reconstruction surgery was, for me, also a no-brainer. And while I lay on my doctor's table that day, thinking about researching reconstruction options and the weighing of those options and the search for a plastic surgeon I would have to undertake in order to make a good swap, I had my first revelation about how I was going to deal with my breast cancer.

As a patient I had been given a diagnosis, and I knew that surgery to remove my breasts lay ahead of me. As a woman, I knew that I was going to want them replaced with very, very good *natural* replicas of the ones I was so very used to caring for and carrying around on a daily basis. It was with the doctor's mind that had been honed in surgical rotations during my medical school education, however, that the patient and the woman I am came to the realization that I had to choose my reconstruction surgeon before I picked anyone else to be on my breast cancer-fighting team.

Why?

Choosing your reconstructive surgeon first is not considered to be the politically correct approach to creating a cancer treatment team. It might seem to some people sort of like picking the ENT to put the tubes in your child's ears before you've seen the pediatrician for the first ear infection. But, with that caveat, hear me out on this one. Have you ever bought a computer? Most of us have purchased several in our lifetimes so we're all fairly familiar with the way a salesperson in a computer store can bombard us with technical information of the sort that only another technician could truly understand—this model comes with 8 MB of storage, 32 MB of storage, potentially unlimited storage if you're using an external drive, but don't confuse memory with hard drive capacity… Oh, *come on*. How many documents does that translate into? How many pages? How many patient files and PowerPoint presentations and research papers can this thing hold? Can I talk to someone who's going to help me visualize my end point? Who can guide me through all my options, all the configurations of all of the components, so that when I walk out of this store I know I'm taking home a computer that will meet my needs.

As a cancer patient, you will have to configure your cancer-fighting team. Your radiologist is concerned with the imaging—the x-rays and mammograms and ultrasounds and other imaging tests—that both provide your diagnosis and guide your medical team in your treatment. Your general surgeon—the doctor who is going to perform your mastectomy—is primarily concerned about removing cancerous tissue from your body. Your oncologist is going to focus on the chemotherapy and/or radiation treatments that might be done prior to your surgery or might follow it. Your breast cancer navigator—often a nurse practitioner and almost always a godsend; a more recently added role in the breast cancer scene that we'll discuss in more detail later—interacts chiefly with these members of the cancer-fighting team to coordinate the multidisciplinary care breast cancer treatment requires. It is your plastic surgeon, however, who is going to reconstruct your breasts—and who is therefore in the best position to help you visualize the end goal: the breasts you will take home at the end of the cancer ordeal.

And why is *that*?

Back to computers. Have you ever bought one only to find that in the next few months it has become outdated? Or that a model more suitable to your needs was actually on the market at the time you made your purchase, but the salesman in your computer store had a bias toward one brand over another? Or maybe he didn't even know about the availability of a feature that would have served you well? The development of new techniques and technologies for breast reconstruction change and improve as rapidly as does computer technology. Bluntly, some general surgeons don't keep up as well as others with the developments in breast reconstruction that would allow them to best serve the desires of their patients; they don't have the time or inclination to get themselves trained in the newest techniques of breast removal that can allow the plastic surgeon to step into the operating room after a mastectomy and do the most artful reconstruction possible. Is, for example, your breast cancer the type for which a nipple-sparing mastectomy is appropriate? Is the general surgeon well practiced in the technique of nipple-sparing surgery? Will he or she work in collaboration with the plastic surgeon to assure that enough tissue has been spared so that the reconstruction can take place as planned? Will your general surgeon cooperate with immediate reconstruction if that's what you want? Your choice of a breast reconstruction surgeon is paramount, as a good one will have worked with a variety of general surgeons and can refer you to one who will collaborate most knowledgeably, and skillfully, toward your end goal.

❧

In order to understand breast cancer,
you first have to understand breasts.
They are the most defining feature of
gender. No other sex characteristic
of either gender is in such plain
view, every day. Even men's most
defining feature, well, that's certainly
not something you see as you
walk down the street everyday, so
even the penis, which has been
invested with so much cultural
baggage, can't be as equally
complex an emotional subject for
men as breasts are for women.

Ankit Desai, M.D.

Julie was a new patient, a southern lady, a real steel magnolia. The first time I met her, for our first consultation, she had very distinct ideas about what sort of reconstruction surgery she wanted and how it was going to work. She told me what technique I was going to use to make her post-surgery breasts look *exactly like* her pre-surgery breasts even before we could talk about the location or stage of her specific cancer.

Most doctors will tell you that they like to work with an informed patient, a patient who can participate really knowledgeably in the decisions the two of you have to make for her health—certainly, I do. But the type of reconstruction options that are available to any one, particular cancer patient depends on a whole host of factors, such as the aforementioned location and stage of the cancer. Before I see a patient, it is very common that she's spent some time on the computer researching breast reconstruction, but often the sites that talk about the individual techniques neglect to go into much detail about the nuances that might make the technique they are recommending a better or worse choice for that one, particular individual.

The problem with such research is that very few of us take the time to educate ourselves about a disease before we actually have it. And then when we're in the middle of a potentially life-threatening health crisis, we're not always in the best frame of mind to absorb and process information. More problematic, in the case of breast cancer, is that breast cancer is an extremely emotional issue from almost every angle—it can be life-threatening as well as *identity*-threatening. Presumably you, the reader, are much like the rest of us in that you've turned to this book for information about breast cancer because you actually have it. Before we talk about treatment options, and the nuances that will help you to have a truly informed and productive discussion with your surgeons—both general and reconstruction—Julie and I want to spend a few pages on some background information that will help you form the questions you'll need to ask, and then evaluate your surgeon's answers.

Basic Breast Anatomy

The mature female breast is a complex structure, and its basic physiology is not as well understood as many may imagine. Outwardly, the breast is an orb—to use a favorite word of Renaissance poets and romance novelists—punctuated by a nipple surrounded by the darker skin of the areola. It is primarily composed of fat—a greater or lesser amount of which determines its size—and connective tissue, a sort of "scaffold" that acts as a mechanical support for other tissues and through which blood vessels and nerve tissue travel. Connective tissue, though the phrase may sound general and somewhat bland, is ubiquitous throughout the human body, a critical component of nearly every organ. Its principal function is as the site of inflammation, the body's first-line defense against injury and invading organisms. Together, the fat and connective tissue are

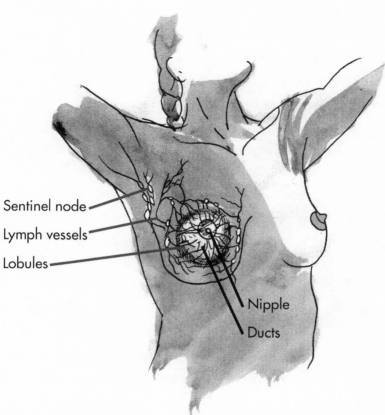

The mature female breast is a complex structure.

known as *stromata,* a word used to distinguish framework tissue from the tissues that perform the specialized function of an organ or gland or other physiological structure. Within the breast there is also a network of arteries and capillaries that carry oxygen and nutrients to the breast tissues, as well as a network of lymph ducts. The lymphatic system is a web of ducts whose function is to fight infection, and to trap toxins and drain them from the body through the lymph nodes that are located all over our bodies, but specifically for the breast, in the armpit and behind the breastbone. There is no muscle tissue in the breasts, though they lie upon a layer of muscle that separates them from the ribs.

Each breast also, of course, contains the components that allow for lactation—lobes and lobules, alveoli and milk ducts—and it is these structures that are the subject of some recent research, and rethinking. Our conventional understanding of the lactating structure of the breast has been based on research done by Sir Astley Cooper[20] in the 1840s and has, surprisingly, considering the vast amount of medical knowledge accumulated since that time, changed little in the one hundred and sixty or so years since he completed his studies. For example, we have known for a long time that the breast contains lobules, or glands, that group together in larger units called lobes, and that the lobes branch out from the nipple, linked by a network of thin tubes or ducts, toward hollow sacs called alveoli. But Sir Astley noted that each breast contained fifteen to twenty lobes, and that these lobes radiated from the nipple in a sunburst, or wheel-spoke pattern. His observations, however, were based on dissection and wax casts. In studies conducted circa 2004-2007, using modern ultrasound imaging,[21] it has been found that the breast contains far fewer lobes—an average of four to eigh-

---

20 Sir Astley Cooper, *On the Anatomy of the Breast*, 1840.

21 http://www.ncbi.nlm.nih.gov/pubmed/17983992.

teen—and that the arrangement of the lobes is more random than the phrase "wheel spoke" would indicate.

Additionally, one of the more recent findings is that researchers were *unable to find* the "lactiferous sinuses" that for nearly two centuries have been thought to be located directly beneath the nipple and act as reservoirs for milk. Ultrasound reveals that the number, size, and shape of these structures are smaller than previously believed, and that their main function may be the transport rather than the storage of milk.[22] Among the clinical implications of this finding is that the importance currently assigned to the positioning and attachment of the baby during breastfeeding may need to be revised.

Breasts, as any woman will attest who has experienced the breast tenderness that often accompanies menstruation, are exquisitely sensitive to cyclical hormonal changes. At puberty it is estrogen, along with progesterone, that triggers breast development and then, after menopause, when the body's production of estrogen decreases, hormones are what trigger the lobes to shrink, or *involute*. When the lobes shrink, they are replaced by fat—a physical swap that accounts for the breasts becoming softer and losing their support as we age. This is why, incidentally, breast size can increase as a woman matures: the breasts of younger women are made up of mostly glandular tissue with little fat, but when the fat content of the breast

---

22 D.T. Ramsay, J.C. Kent, R.A. Owens, P.E. Hartmann, "Ultrasound Imaging of Milk Ejection in the Breast of Lactating Women," *Pediatrics* **113** (2), 2004, 361–367.

increases through the shrinkage of the lobes, the breasts are then as prone as other areas of the body to react to fluctuations in weight.

In relation to cancer, one factor of the physiology of the breast that is essential to note is the difference in consistencies between two key components of the breast: the lobes and the fat. The lobes, or the glandular portion of the breast, have a firm, nodular texture, while the fat is soft. When conducting a breast exam, many women believe they or their doctor are feeling for "lumps," but what the careful palpation of the breast should actually reveal is the difference in consistencies between the lobes and the fat. This is why monthly self-breast examinations are so important: a woman should become familiar with the feel of the nodules in her own breasts and be able to detect changes in them that indicate further examination by a physician is required. Additionally, one is generally unable to feel the ducts within the glandular portion of the breast unless one is lactating, or a duct is inflamed or contains a tumor. Why is this key? *Because most breast cancers begin in the ducts, some in the cells that line the lobes, and only a small percentage in other breast tissues.*

Similarly, the technology behind the mammogram relies on the differences in densities between fat and glandular breast tissue. Mammograms—*annual* mammograms—are so critical, however, because they detect changes in the breast that cannot be felt but show up only on the breast x-ray films. The changes that show up on mammograms are called *calcifications*. Breast calcifications—small clusters of calcium in breast tissue—are

AGE AT WHICH BREAST CANCER IS DIAGNOSED

It was estimated in 2010 that 207,090 women would be diagnosed with breast cancer before the year was out.[1]

In the years between 2004 and 2008, the median age at which a woman was diagnosed was sixty-one.

There were not a statistically significant number of cases of breast cancer in women under twenty.

- 1.9% of the cases of breast cancer occurred in women between the ages of twenty and thirty-four.

- 10.2% of the cases of breast cancer occurred in women between the ages of thirty-five and forty-four.

- 22.6% in women who were between the ages forty-five and fifty-four.

- 24.4% between the ages of fifty-five and sixty-four.

- 19.7% between sixty-five and seventy-four.

- 15.5% between seventy-five and eighty-four.

- 5.6% for women eighty-five years and older.[2]

1 http://seer.cancer.gov/statfacts/html/breast.html.

2 Ibid.

fairly common, and most are harmless. There are two types of them: macrocalcifications and microcalcifications.

Macrocalcifications are grainy deposits that show up rather like the dots and dashes of Morse code on a mammogram film. They're not caused by dietary sources of calcium, drinking milk or eating ice cream or taking calcium supplements, but may be the result of a previous inflammation or injury, or simply the result of aging. Approximately half of women who are over fifty can expect that some macrocalcifications will turn up in a mammogram, versus only about ten percent of younger women. They are harmless, and require no additional monitoring.

Microcalcifications are, as their name suggests, smaller calcium deposits that show up as white flecks on a mammogram film. They are usually an indication that in the specific area of the breast, cells are being replaced at a more rapid-than-normal rate. A microcalcification is not necessarily an indication of cancer. If one is found on your mammogram, your radiologist will first check the pattern or cluster that the calcification has formed, as certain patterns can imply that cancerous or pre-cancerous cells are present. Depending on the pattern of the microcalcification, your doctor will likely recommend that you have a *magnification mammogram* so she or he can get a more close-up view of the area of concern. Again, depending on what this second mammogram indicates, your doctor may then recommend a biopsy, a diagnostic procedure in which a small sample of tissue is taken from the area of concern and looked at under a microscope.

So what is breast cancer? What is that thing we are hoping not to find under the lens of the microscope? It is a proliferation of cells that start reproducing on an accelerated basis, creating a mass. If unchecked, that mass can propagate, grow larger, and the cancerous cells can travel through the blood stream and the lymphatic system to other areas of the body. If the cancer is caught at an early stage, however, survival rates are excellent. According to the National Cancer Institute, the 5-year survival rate is 98.6%[23] for "localized cancer"—that is, cancer that is detected early and is confined to the primary or original site of occurrence. For "regional" cancer—that is, cancer that has spread to regional lymph nodes—the survival rate is 83.8%.[24] For "distant" cancer, or cancer that has metastasized, the rate is 23.4%.[25]

When should you take the proactive step of beginning to have annual mammograms to screen for breast cancer? At what age? Although official recommendations—and, therefore, what may or may not be covered under an individual's insurance policy—vary, an appropriate and loving fortieth birthday gift to yourself or to any woman you know may well be her first annual mammogram.

---

23 http://seer.cancer.gov/statfacts/html/breast.html.

24 Ibid.

25 Ibid.

Yes, but what *causes* cancer? Injury to genetic material, or genetic mutation. "Cancer results when cells accumulate genetic errors and multiply without control."[26] Well, what causes the genetic error? And how can I help my genes to correct their mistakes? In order to answer those questions, a little more background material is in order.

> Cancer is what happens when
> your body is overwhelmed by a
> cumulative dose of stuff that shouldn't
> be in your body in the first place.
>
> *Julie*

Too often, cancer is viewed from the wrong side of the looking glass: we decide what to do about it only when we are forced to do something about it—only after we actually have it. In our pre-cancer lives we don't think about how we might lower our risks of getting sick, let alone fashion our lives around the preventative measures we might take. I know I didn't, and as a doctor I knew at least as well as anyone else what those measures are. As we said earlier, we all know that smoking is very

---

26 http://ghr.nlm.nih.gov/handbook/illustrations/cancer.

bad for us. It is the underlying cause of a number of deadly cancers and other diseases, and most of us have taken the immeasurably positive step of quitting it, or of not starting in the first place. But the risks associated with smoking have been well publicized for decades and there really is no excuse *not* to know about them. What about the risks associated with any number of other toxins as common today as second-hand smoke was back in 1963? And, beyond eliminating risk, what of proactive, preventative things we can *add* to our daily routines to keep our all-too-human bodies from getting sick? How much do we really know about these things?

In this book, we're going to look at cancer through the lens of *functional medicine*. Functional medicine is a branch of medicine that deals with disease prevention, and with tackling the causes that underlie serious, chronic disease rather than merely treating the symptoms—that is, while the doctors were busy *curing* my cancer with the time-honored treatments and techniques of traditional, Western medicine, I got busy dealing with and correcting the reasons I *got* cancer by putting into practice the findings of a whole different and newer branch of science: Functional Medicine.

Functional medicine has six core principles:

1. Each individual human being has a unique biochemistry—a totally unique mix of the natural human chemical components that sustain life: proteins and carbohydrates, peptides and acids and neurotransmitters and such—and the way that this mix works is dependent on each per-

son's genetic makeup, their personal rate of metabolic function, and the stresses that are specific to the environment in which they live. Further, the "environment" takes into consideration not just the person's physical surroundings—the home and the town in which they reside, and such factors as the quality of the food they are able to put on their table or how close to a toxic waste facility the town is located—but also their emotional environment. Does this person find his job fulfilling? How is that person handling a difficult marital relationship? Functional medicine is not "one size fits all." As a simple example, a doctor who practices functional medicine may recommend that, in general, a full-grown man or woman supplement his or her diet with 5,000 units of vitamin D daily; for a lifeguard who spends eight hours a day sitting in the sun, soaking up the sun's vitamin D, the doctor may well decrease this dosage.

2. Patient care is given weight over disease care. Sir William Osler was one of the four founding professors of Johns Hopkins Hospital and the creator of the first residency program for the specialty training of physicians, taking them out of the lecture hall and putting them by the bedsides of real patients in order to learn. Functional medicine takes its lead from Osler's tenet that "It is more important to know what patient has the disease than to know what disease the patient has." Let's illustrate this with an example from fashion. There is, in the window of my local women's dress shop, a really cute orange sun-dress. It has a skinny tank top and a short, flippy skirt and, as an accent at the waistband, a big yellow fabric daisy. It is an absolutely adorable piece of clothing but, because I am a sensible middle-aged woman, when I go into the store to buy the dress, I don't ask for it in my size, I ask for it in my daughter's. A dress is not a dress is not a dress; what is suitable for one age and lifestyle is a disaster for another. When it comes to disease, successful treatment can be greatly enhanced by taking into consideration factors such as the patient's age, general health, lifestyle and activity level.

3. The body's biochemical balance is dynamic, and to achieve an optimal one, one must take into consideration changing internal and external factors. Pretend that you are standing on a block of flat wood that is resting on top of a circular log; your job is to stay balanced on that piece of wood. Whether you can do it or not is based on inter-nal factors—what you're doing with your muscles to keep from falling off that block of wood—as well as on exter-nal forces such as, let's say, a sixty-mile-an-hour wind gusting up. Maintaining your balance on top of that block of wood depends on the interaction between your muscles contracting so you can lean into the wind (inter-nal factor) and the wind itself (which is external)—and it depends as well on how you adapt when the internal or external factors change, when your thigh muscle cramps, or the wind dies down, or someone pushes you. In a similar fashion, what your body needs each day to stay in balance is always changing. For example, your body's need for vitamin C changes on a daily basis. Among the benefits of vitamin C is that it is a great antioxidant so, for that reason alone, it should be part of anyone's daily supplement routine. But if you are in a situation where your oxidative stress is increased—you are pulling an all-nighter to get ready for a big presentation the next day or you're getting sick—your body's need for vitamin C also increases. There is no resting on your laurels, so to speak, when it comes to maintaining your health. Life and the situations in life that we all encounter along the way are not static, and therefore neither are the things, such as nutrients and exercise, for example, that your body requires to efficiently and energetically meet the always-changing challenges of normal human life.

4. The body is a symphonic machine. As one could not play Beethoven's Fifth without all of the instruments for which it is scored—or, at least, it would not really be Beethoven's Fifth without a timpani and a piccolo player among the musicians—all of the instruments, all of the organs and other structures of the human body, must work in concert for the whole body to perform with a truly harmonious vitality. Dietary deficits can cause neurological problems, environmental insults can cause hormonal dysfunctions, and such a simple thing as not

flossing your teeth can contribute to cardiovascular disease. Even more plainly: what you put into your stomach influences how well your brain works; how close you live to a coal-burning power plant could impact on your ability to have a baby; you could start every day by running five miles, but if you don't care for your smile you are not doing all you can to keep your heart healthy.

5. Health is not merely the absence of disease. That is, health can't be described in the negative—it is a positive attribute. Let's say that you're taking a class at your local college. It's a class in advanced accounting that you need in order to get ahead at the office, or a class in American history you're taking simply because you always wanted to know more about the subject. To pass the class, all you need to do is to get a C. But all a C means is that you've done the minimum amount of work, and absorbed the minimum amount of knowledge that you need to skate by. Striving for an A, however, means that you've got to really apply yourself to the task, and at the end of it your knowledge of accounting or American history will be more robust than if you settle for the so-so C. As abundance is not merely the absence of poverty, or happiness is not merely the absence of sadness, being truly healthy is not a matter of skating by, content that you aren't sick; it is not a matter of shuffling through the race, but of being able to approach the race with vitality and enough reserve to be able to run it with vigor.

6. Promotion of organ reserve enhances health span. The phrase "organ reserve" refers to the ability of our organs to sustain and support life. When we are children, our organs have the capacity to do much more work than our young bodies require them to do. This is one of the reasons that young people can bounce back from sickness and injury more quickly than those of us who are older. As we age—encounter repeated illness or injury and contend with the cumulative effects of poor diet and lack of exercise and exposure to environmental toxins such as the pesticides used to grow the bulk of the foods offered in our supermarkets—our organs are repeatedly pushed to the limits of their capacity, and the reserves we enjoyed as children begin to diminish. Our organs, therefore, begin to do their jobs under stress—but there are things that we can do to alleviate, and even reverse that stress. Since I've used the example of supplements frequently in this section, let's stay with the vitamin theme and illustrate what I'm talking about here with the "daily value" that gets printed on the labels of many vitamin brands. This daily value is not what your body needs in order to function optimally; it is merely the minimum daily dose required in order for you to avoid manifesting a deficiency disease state. And this daily dose changes from day to day. Think money, for a moment. Think of the minimum amount of it you need every week to shelter and feed and clothe your family. If that minimum amount that you need is also the maximum amount you earn, then there is never

an opportunity to put any money in the bank to have it waiting there securely for a rainy day; there is no extra, no reserve. Moreover, the minimum amount you need changes from day to day. The bills are higher in the winter when the heater runs than they are in the summer when you can open all of the windows and live comfortably. Your body needs more nutrients than it minimally requires so that it—so that your organs—can build up and securely maintain a reserve of health to use for a rainy day.

If we look at human health through the lens of functional medicine, with an understanding that health can't be "compartmentalized"—that is, the heart and the liver and the brain and the breast don't work separately from each other to create and sustain life any more than the timpani or the piccolo can create and sustain a symphony all by itself—an interesting way to look at disease emerges: *disease*, by whatever name we call it—autism or Alzheimer's, heart disease or breast cancer—is, at its root, a problem of cells that are malfunctioning somewhere in the body. In fact, Bob Rountree, MD, a functional medicine practitioner and Institute for Functional Medicine faculty member, has gone so far as to say that when we understand that the body is truly restorative, we have to also understand that there really is no such thing as disease, only a failure of the body to restore itself. The challenge, then, in both healing and preventing disease, is to get and to keep our cells at their optimum performance levels.

Taking on cancer from the perspective of functional medicine does not, however, mean that we bypass the treatments that traditional, Western medicine offers. Not by a long shot. I love the general surgeon who cut the cancer from my body, and I love the oncologist whose energy-sapping, intravenous chemicals made my hair fall out, and I really adore the gifted surgeon, my coauthor, who so artfully used the cutting edge technologies and techniques developed by innovative traditional practitioners and researchers to reconstruct my breasts after my mastectomies. They were all a critical part of my cancer-fighting team. But while the surgeon and the oncologist were cutting out and poisoning the cancer, I was hard at work detoxifying myself, improving the quality of my biochemical makeup, and taking part in a whole host of other non-traditional, science-based therapies that vastly improved my cancer-survival odds and enabled me to function through my treatments with less pain, faster healing, and more vitality. The functional-medicine piece balances the traditional Western-medicine methods of beating cancer, and enhances them so that the cancer becomes, biologically, a much more beatable foe. It restores the body's unique, biological equilibrium, so that the cancer, once beaten, thinks twice about coming back for another showdown. And by incorporating the healthy habits, supplements and practices that are at the core of functional medicine, people who have yet to be sidelined by a major disease like cancer may greatly increase their chances of avoiding such world-rocking sickness altogether.

All right. So now that you have some basic background information about the lens through which we are looking at cancer, let's go back to that question about genetic errors. What causes these errors? It starts with the aluminum in your deodorant. The mercury you come into contact with, whether directly, such as the mercury in most dental fillings, or indirectly, such as the mercury that is released from your area's coal-burning power plant. The BPAs in your plastic water bottle. The pesticides in your food, and the residue of pesticides in your cotton clothing. The electromagnetic radiation coming off your phone, the router in your house, the HD television, the wireless keyboard, the wireless house phone handsets. The chemicals in your hair dye and makeup and fingernail polish. In cleaning products and weed killers. In carpets and couches and beds that have been manufactured using a chemical process. It starts with the exhaust fumes swirling around your car as you creep through stop-and-go traffic on the freeway, late for a meeting, beeping your horn, checking your watch, punching at your cell phone, sending a text, cursing out the driver who cut you off and who cursed you right back because he is late and all stressed out, too.

These constant, common, cumulative insults to your biological system manifest in the oxidative stress and chronic inflammation I detailed in the last chapter, the two big culprits in the cause of disease. And the oxidative stress and chronic inflammation can cause a variety of other fundamental physiological dysfunctions. According to the Institute for Functional Medicine,[27] these are:

1. Hormonal and neurotransmitter imbalances (most easily understood if we think about the widely acknowledged negative impact of chronically elevated stress hormones like cortisol and adrenaline)

2. Oxidation-reduction imbalances and mitochondropathy (which is oxidative stress and dysfunction of the mitochondria—the energy synthesizers of our cells)

3. Detoxification and biotransformational imbalances (which means your body develops trouble in carrying out the natural, vital task of ridding itself of the toxic compounds, such as heavy metals and other chemicals, with which it comes into contact)

4. Immune imbalances (loss of the very delicate balance between the types of immune responses your body makes all day, every day to the environment we create for it)

5. Inflammatory imbalances (which is that chronic inflammatory response and closely related to immune responses)

---

27 http://www.functionalmedicine.org/about/whatis.asp.

6. Digestive, absorptive, and microbiological imbalances (loss of the balance of microbes and enzymes that flourish in a healthy gut that is fed with true food rather than processed junk)

7. Structural imbalances from cellular membrane function to the musculoskeletal system (disruption of the building blocks that make up our cell membranes, or disruption of the fundamental structure of our larger organ systems, like our muscles, or our nerves, or our skeleton)

But there is one other typical, modern medical dysfunction that can result from the cumulative effects of living a typical, modern, stress- and chemical-filled life: your body's *methylation* system can go awry. When this happens—when the daily environmental insults progress to the level of methylation interference—the real trouble begins.

Methylation is a complex biochemical process that can be explained somewhat simply: a group of atoms (the "methyl group" that consists of one carbon and three hydrogen atoms) are added or subtracted to or from a molecule within a cell. But while swapping out a few atoms can sound unassuming, this is a process that goes on thousands of times every day in every cell of your body and is simply essential to life. The processes that healthy methylation promotes in the body are myriad, and though we know a great deal about it, science has likely not yet discovered all of its beneficial functions.

One benefit we know about for sure is that efficient methylation is key in enhancing the function of serotonin. Serotonin is a neurotransmitter and, among the amazing functions that it allows our body to accomplish are the regulation of the digestive tract, bone growth and bone density, and mood. When the body doesn't produce enough serotonin, we may end up with diarrhea, osteoporosis, and depression. And, without

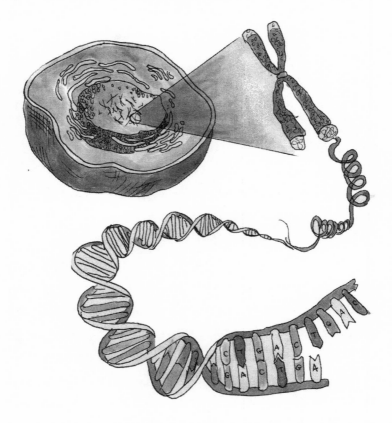

DNA takes the shape of a double helix. Healthy DNA remains tightly packed within the cell. When DNA is damaged and unpacks it sends the wrong messages to the body, including, "Make cancer."

efficient methylation, our body's use of serotonin can't be optimized in preventing these health problems.

Methylation is also foundational to the production of melatonin, a hormone that helps to regulate our circadian rhythms or, more simply, our response to light and dark, sunlight and nighttime. Dysfunctional methylation = lower melatonin production = difficulty falling asleep or staying asleep.

Methylation is critical to the body's natural detox system too—it is a trigger that initiates cellular reaction to the presence of a toxicant in the body, "instructing" the cells to capture the poison and drain it from the body—and it is critical as well to the control of homocysteine levels. Homocysteine is an amino acid, and elevated levels of it have been linked to cardiovascular disease, Alzheimer's, depression, liver disease, and accelerated aging.

Last, and perhaps most important of all, when our body is not methylating properly, the dysfunction decreases the natural production of *glutathione*. Glutathione is a peptide that we will talk about in more detail later in this book; for now, let it suffice to say that it is the body's master antioxidant; of all of the naturally occurring biochemicals our body manufactures to control oxidative stress, and of all the dietary supplements such as vitamin C that we can take to combat free radicals, none are more effective than the body's own good, old glutathione. Too low a level of methylation means less glutathione means more oxidative stress—and, in a sort of circular, symphonic irony, more oxidative stress causes lower levels of methylation. *The body is a symphonic machine*; as the piccolo and the timpani need to work together to produce the full orchestration the composer intended, the processes of the body need to work together or the vibrant health that is possible cannot be achieved.

When the body is methylating at a substandard rate, the condition is called *hypomethylation*. When the hypomethylation is not addressed and corrected and so continues for a long period of time, that condition is known as *chronic hypomethylation*. Chronic hypomethylation of your DNA is the mechanism by which diseases, like cancer, take hold.

Most of us know that our DNA takes the shape of a double helix, two smooth, three-dimensional curves similar to the coils of a mattress spring or the red and blue of the barbershop pole winding around each other in perfect symmetry. What we might not know is that within the cell, the DNA is very tightly packed. And at the end of this tightly packed DNA, there are telomeres—big, thick, strong telomeres that guard the DNA, ensuring that it stays coiled tightly, much like keeping the lid on an old-fashioned Jack-in-the-Box. Hypomethylation has *two* negative effects on our DNA, that's how important it is to methylate well! The first negative effect is to allow our telomeres to shorten, to become weak and ineffective at keeping the DNA tightly packed, at keeping the lid on the Jack-in-the-Box. The second negative effect is to allow that DNA to unpack and to start expressing itself. Expressing more DNA than a cell needs is sort of a cellular TMI (too much information!) experience. When our DNA becomes unpacked, and the telomeres at the ends of our DNA strands begin to weaken and shorten, it allows the DNA on the chromosome to send several different and grave messages that the body then acts upon—among them, "Age faster," and "Make cancer!"[28] If the telomere suffers enough damage, the gene will mutate—a mutation being a permanent change in the DNA sequence that makes up a gene.

The good news is that it is possible to reverse the damage to the telomeres, and to repack the DNA so it is nice and snug again in its double helix. How do we do this? Through diet, exercise and other therapies that can improve low methylation rates and get them back up to speed.

In the following chapters we outline the diagnostic process for breast cancer, the traditional treatment options that each breast cancer patient must weigh, as well as the treatments and therapies that functional medicine offers to complement them, to speed and enhance recovery and get that DNA cozily packed up once again so it stops sending the "Make cancer!" message.

---

28 http://www.nature.com/nature/journal/v395/n6697/abs/395089a0.html

2

Functional Medicine Approach

The Role of Hyperbarics

'Take a breather.' It's shorthand for stopping to rest, ceasing an activity in order to catch one's breath, taking a deep breath. So intuitively do we know how important it is to simply breathe we've made a cliché of it—but rarely do we stop to think about the wisdom inherent in the cliché, how fundamental oxygen is to our health.

Julie

The kids took the news better than I
could have hoped. My husband and I gathered them in the
family room that first night I knew I had cancer and told
them I was sick, and what they did astonished me. My son,
then fourteen, nodded at us, as is his habit when he wants a
moment to think things over before he speaks; a good trait for
a kid who has decided he wants to be a doctor like his mom
when he grows up—and then he started asking questions. How
big was the cancer? What stage was it? Had I decided yet on a
treatment plan? My husband and I answered these questions
as calmly and thoroughly as we could—even given that what
we had at that point were pretty thin answers—so I suppose it
was simply the idea that his mom was sick that started the tears,
and the tears were contagious: my daughter began next. We
had a good, tight family hug, and a good, calming, cleansing
family cry. It was a necessary, healing moment, and actually
pretty lovely.

Then my son—the future medical student, remember—
got up and went to his room, fired up his computer and sat
down for a long night of Googling around to find out every-

thing he could about breast cancer. My daughter, Dani, however, didn't want to let go of her father and me. She didn't want to stop hugging.

Dani, those who have read my previous book about the biomedical approach to treating autism will know, is herself autistic. One of the symptoms of autism that we first noticed in her was her indifference to human contact—I could leave the house and she wouldn't even know or care if I was gone; I could give her a hug and she would stiffen against my embrace as if it were unwelcome. This indifference was utterly heartbreaking, and persisted through many years of treatment. The evening that, out of the blue, after years of lacking all interest in touching another human being, Dani came over to where I was sitting on the sofa and snuggled herself into my arms— well, that moment remains one of the greatest victories of my life. Needless to say, I did not take for granted her need and desire to hold onto me the night she found out that I was sick. We were sad, but somewhere inside me I was doing a Snoopy Happy Dance: cancer was definitely lemons, but Dani's sympathy and empathy, well, that was some serious lemonade.

Dani's big, tight hug was also an inspiration. Some of our best snuggle time in the last few years had been the nights we'd spent together in our family's hyperbaric chamber. In my office I have two hyperbaric chambers, for my patients' use, and our family has, as the families of many autistic children do, made the investment and purchased one for our home so that Dani would be able to have more access to the healing it provided. But Dani and I hadn't, of late, been able to spend many nights, or even many hours, together in the chamber—other "priorities" of my stress-filled life had gotten in the way. I'd given up much of my time in the chamber in order to service other demands in my life, but this sacrifice hadn't been a service to Dani, who needed the therapy for her illness and didn't especially relish getting into the chamber alone—and, as it turned out, it wasn't a service to me either: hyperbaric therapy helps to heal the effects of stress, oxidative stress and chronic inflammatory response and hypomethylation. All the things that had conspired to cause my cancer.

Moreover, I knew that hyperbaric therapy was not merely a cancer-prevention tool: *hyperbaric therapy can help to heal cancer.*

I turned to my husband, both of us clutched in Dani's warm embrace, and said, "Would you mind if I get into the chamber with Dani?"

My husband smiled. "I think that's a terrific idea."

Hyperbaric therapy, or hyperbaric oxygen therapy (HBOT) is, essentially, the medical use of plain, old oxygen, albeit under higher atmospheric pressure than is possible by simply breathing. I have successfully used it with my autistic patients, my injured NFL players, menopausal mothers and my elder patients who refer to it as "the fountain of youth." I had routinely advised my patients' parents, those intrepid caregivers, to crawl into the chamber with their children at every possible opportunity as the therapy helps not only our young, primary patients, but their caregivers in stress modulation—and I suspect, since this is something I've observed over many years of use in my office, that it may decrease addictive drives for substances such as alcohol, tobacco, and other drugs, which is a key component of stress management as stress also increases the desire to indulge in addictive substances. Now I was going to use it as a tool in my fight against breast cancer.

The word hyperbaric means, literally, "high" (hyper) "pressure" (baric). And though just beginning to emerge in mainstream medicine as a go-to therapeutic tool for a variety of seemingly unrelated illnesses, it has been around for centuries. Its most likely father was a British clergyman named Henshaw who, in 1662, constructed an entire room to act as a chamber in which air pressure could be increased by use of an organ bellows. The increased air pressure, he believed, could help people who suffered from acute pulmonary, or lung-related, ailments, among other illnesses. This was the same year, it should be noted, that physicist and chemist Robert Boyle first published his law, known now as Boyle's Law, describing the relationship between pressure and gas. Simply stated, Boyle discovered that pressure decreases the volume of gas or, in other words, condenses it. Henshaw's enormous hyperbaric "device," however, increased only air pressure, but did not directly increase the concentration of oxygen. It wasn't until 1772 that chemists Carl Wilhelm Scheele, a Swede, and Joseph Priestly, who was English, isolated the element of oxygen and real advances in the science of hyperbarics began.

Over the centuries, in both Europe and North America, hyperbaric therapy was used to treat cholera, rickets, nervous disorders, diabetes, syphilis, and the victims of the Spanish

Influenza epidemic that swept the United States at the close of WWI. It wasn't until the mid-1930s, however, when the use of hyperbarics proved effective in the treatment of decompression sickness in deep sea divers, that the U.S. military took notice of its benefits, and its potential uses for military purposes. That's when the age of modern hyperbarics really began.

Hyperbaric therapy is based on a simple fact: breathing—*air*—is essential to life. We breathe because cells that are deprived of oxygen will die. Normally, however, the air that we breathe is composed of about 21% oxygen. Modern hyperbarics works by allowing us to breathe up to 100% oxygen, both condensing the gas and pressurizing it so that it penetrates our blood stream at a much higher and faster rate than is possible in any other circumstance. In our blood stream, the oxygen binds to the hemoglobin in our red blood cells—which is the standard way the element is carried to our tissues and organs—but, when under pressure, it also dissolves into our plasma. Plasma is the thin, yellowish fluid in which our blood cells are transported throughout the body, carrying air and nutrients and other life-giving essentials to all the rest of our cells. This dissolved oxygen, which is, with hyperbarics, so much more plentiful in the blood stream, can penetrate deep into our tissues and organs, flooding damaged cells with the healing element. Flooding the brains of children who have cerebral palsy with oxygen has been shown to reawaken dormant areas of the brain,[29]—

---

29 *http://www.thelancet.com/journals/lancet/article/*
PIIS0140-6736(00)05136-9/fulltext.

and, by the same principle, hyperbarics may offer new hope for stroke victims, no matter how long ago their strokes may have occurred.[30] Flooding the injuries of my bruised and battered NFL players with oxygen after a game has reduced inflammation and swelling as well as the actual physical appearance of hematomas as the extra oxygen breaks down the unsightly bruise itself and carries away the crusted blood and other cells via the blood stream. Flooding my autistic patients with oxygen, of course, seems to improve every system in their little bodies—improving immune function, facilitating digestion and improving other gut problems, and helping to clear the "autistic fog" that makes them present as if their intellectual and emotional capacities are lesser than those of neurotypical children; in short, addressing and improving, simultaneously and painlessly, every symptom of autism.

In the case of cancer, however, I think hyperbarics has a profound additional benefit.

In 1931, Otto Heinrich Warburg won the Nobel Prize in Physiology and Medicine for his work on the respiration of cells and the metabolism of tumors. *Metabolism* is a set of chemical reactions that happen within living cells to sustain life—reactions that allow the cells to maintain their structural integrity and to grow, to respond to what is happening in their environment, and to reproduce. There are two types of metabolism: *catabolism*, which, as we've mentioned earlier,

---

30 http://www.calgaryhyperbariccentre.com/docs/Hyperbaric_Oxygenation_
Adjunct_Therapy_in_Strokes_due_to_Thrombosis.pdf.

is the breaking down of organic matter such as food and diet supplements; and *anabolism*, which is the process of constructing the biochemicals, such as proteins and nucleic acids, that our bodies need to function.

What Warburg found out was that the metabolic process for cancer cells is diametrically different than the metabolic process of normal adult cells—and, for many years, this difference was thought to be the *result* of tumor development, not the *cause*. But as science has progressed, we are discovering that, in fact, Warburg was really on to something;[31] in the last couple of years, cancer research has begun to focus new treatment approaches on this difference in metabolism.

So, what is this difference? Normal adult cells use the *mitochondria*—the tiny "energy factories" inside our cells—to produce their energy needs using oxygen. This is an *aerobic* process, meaning that it requires air in order to take place. Think of the term we all know, "aerobic exercise," which refers to sustained activities such as running or playing basketball that use air in the energy-generating process within the muscles, versus "anaerobic exercise," such as weight lifting, in which muscle energy is generated through tension, or short bursts of high-intensity activity.

Cancer cells rely on the anaerobic process to sustain their life, to replicate, and to spread. Physiologically, this anaerobic

---

31 http://www.xuyue.net/pub/wenxian/%BF%B9%D2%A9%D0%D4%BA%C
D%B9%CC%CC%E5%D6%D7%C1%F6%CE%A2%BB%B7%BE%B3/On%20
the%20Origin%20of%20Cancer%20Cells.pdf.

process is called *glycolysis*, referring to the fact that cancer cells derive their energy from glucose, or sugar, and—here is the key part—*cancer cells will rely on glycolysis even when oxygen is available to them*. The *only* way that cancer cells sustain their lives, and grow at the accelerated rate that they do, is via their unique metabolic process.[32]

So, what does this tell us about the therapeutic benefits of providing an oxygen-rich environment for our cells when we have been given a diagnosis of cancer? Within the traditional medical community, the jury is still out. In a nod to this traditional thinking, let me concede that I have here greatly condensed the complex science behind "the Warburg Effect," which is that cancer cells continue to rely on glycolysis even in the presence of oxygen, and that more research is wanted in order to settle a hotly debated topic: is glycolysis the cause of cancer or a by-product of it?[33] But let me also point out that there is often a crucial gap between what is proven in a laboratory and what works in clinical practice. What we can say for sure is that on-going research tells us cancer cells do not flourish in an oxygen-rich environment.[34]

---

32 *http://www.sciencedaily.com/releases/2008/03/080312141243.htm*; *http://www.ncbi.nlm.nih.gov/pubmed/18337823*; http://www.ncbi.nlm.nih.gov/pubmed/18337815.

33 http://jnci.oxfordjournals.org/content/96/24/1805.full.

34 A few scholarly articles on the benefits of hyperbaric therapy in fighting cancer: *http://www.thelancet.com/journals/lancet/article/PIIS0140-6736(77)90116-7/abstract*; *http://www.springerlink.com/content/wg82q0021741335g/*; http://www.nejm.org/doi/full/10.1056/NEJM199606203342506.

And hyperbaric therapy saturates the cells within our bodies with oxygen.

Diving into the hyperbaric chamber with Dani that first night—and many nights thereafter throughout my cancer ordeal—was most definitely a, "Well, *duh*" moment.

Duh having been uttered, however, it is important to draw a clear distinction between what we are talking about in this chapter—hyperbaric therapy, or HBOT—and what is generally referred to as "oxygen therapy." In HBOT, the patient essentially takes a leisurely nap in—or, at low pressures, even spends the night sleeping comfortably in—an enclosed chamber filled with pressurized air. The chamber is about the same dimensions as the lower bunk in a set of bunk beds, and the downsides are few:

- **Some people may feel discomfort** in their ears or sinuses as the chamber comes up to pressure, similar to the way some people feel in a plane upon takeoff or landing, and this is easily countered by the same tricks that fliers and divers employ to equalize their eardrums—swallowing, or holding the nose and blowing gently.

- **You should avoid wearing perfumes** or colognes into the chamber as the scents, pleasant enough in a normal atmosphere, can become quite intense and often unpleasant under pressure.

● **You should make sure to hit the bathroom** before you
dive into the hyperbaric chamber—the pressure in the
"tank" helps all of the fluids that accumulate in your legs
during the day to go straight back to your kidneys, filling
your bladders in a hurry. I often try to put my feet up for
an hour before getting in the chamber for the evening,
hoping to make it all night before I've got to go to the
bathroom.

● **It can get chilly inside the chamber**—not cold, but
crisp—and so I always make sure I take a nice, soft blanket in with me.

"Oxygen therapy" is quite a bit different from HBOT. It is
generally an invasive procedure in which hydrogen peroxide
or ozone is introduced into the body via injection into muscle
tissue or blood stream, or even through the rectum or vagina.
Such therapies are controversial, at best, and they may even be
dangerous. Oxygen therapy certainly was outside of my comfort zone when I was looking at treatment options.

That said, there are, however, a few circumstances under
which you may want or need to avoid HBOT. Pregnant
women have been advised to forego hyperbarics, more because
there isn't published research on its use in this situation than
because it's known to be a risk or a problem. In fact, the consensus is clearly that it should be used if a person suffers smoke
inhalation and carbon monoxide exposure, pregnant or not.
Insulin-dependent diabetics must monitor their sugars very

carefully when using hyperbarics, and anyone who has had a recent pneumothorax should avoid chamber use. My textbook said that those taking certain drugs such as Antabuse for the treatment of alcoholism should not use hyperbarics, although I've never found an explanation of why this might be. In relation to cancer, specifically, there has been discussion on the web of avoiding hyperbarics when using certain chemotherapeutic agents, such as Adriamycin and Cisplatin. Suggestions were made, in the form of an abstract by John J. Feldmeier, DO in 2009, at an Annual Science Meeting of the Undersea and Hyperbaric Medical Society,[35] not because of known drug interactions or unacceptable side effects, but because the mode of action of these particular chemo agents is more or less "opposite" to the mode of action of oxygen in the body, and the assumption was made that they probably shouldn't be used together. It was suggested that, at the least, hyperbarics can safely be resumed when the course of chemotherapy is complete.

It is important to understand, as we think about oxygen, hyperbarics, and cancer, that Dr. Feldmeier has published extensively in the medical literature on using hyperbaric therapy to counter the side effects of radiation therapy. In 2003, he published a paper reviewing what we knew about hyperbarics and whether it promoted growth or recurrence of malignancy. His conclusion was that there was little basis in the medical

---

35 http://archive.rubicon-foundation.org/xmlui/handle/123456789/9124

literature to suggest that hyperbaric oxygen would enhance malignant growth or metastases.[36]

What you want to look for in a hyperbaric therapy facility is one that offers *low-pressure* hyperbaric chambers, or "mild personal" or "soft shell" hyperbaric chambers. High-pressure chambers, the original design and function of the therapy, are hard-shelled, made of metal, deliver oxygen under an amount of pressure that can itself be stressful to the body, and the sessions can be terribly expensive—around $1200 per hour! Advancements in the understanding of how hyperbarics works have led to the development of low-pressure, soft-sided chambers, such as the ones I use in my office and have at home. These personal chambers, when inflated, look like a long tube, and are about the width of a camp cot. They fit two adults fairly comfortably—and are ideal for parent and child!—delivering life-giving oxygen at a pressure that nourishes and pleases the body's tissues, all at an average cost of about $100 per hour.

Please see the Resources section at the end of this book for help in finding a hyperbaric therapy facility near you, or to rent or purchase your own hyperbaric chamber for in-home use. Meantime, writing this chapter has inspired me—I am going to go look for Dani and see if she wants to curl up in the chamber with me for an hour or so.

When you have finished your cancer treatments, and come out on the other side of your cancer ordeal, consider continuing regular sessions in a hyperbaric chamber. We need oxygen

---

36 http://www.ncbi.nlm.nih.gov/pubmed/12841604.

not just to help heal us when we're sick but to *maintain* optimal physical health and mental clarity—and slash the chances that our cancer will recur. How much hyperbaric therapy is enough—and how much is too much? The good news is that there is no "end point" to the benefits of hyperbarics—the more oxygen your cells receive, the better they like it. During the treatment phase of my cancer experience, I spent a minimum of two nights a week, or a total of sixteen hours a week, in the chamber. I was fascinated by how it helped to relieve my chemo-associated nausea. These days, I like to get at least one night or eight hours in the chamber a week, but I know that what we'd like to make happen and what is possible are not always the same thing and I don't add to my daily stress level by becoming undone when I can't get what I'd like. I am religious only about maintaining a minimum of two one-hour sessions a week. Remember: good health is not the opposite of disease—it is a whole other thing entirely; it is vitality, enthusiasm, presence, not only willingness to approach the race with good intentions, but the ability to run the race with gusto! Then remember that running is an intensely aerobic exercise—give your body the fuel, the oxygen, it needs to complete any race that you decide to enter.

3

Detection and Diagnosis

Hi, Mary, do you do breast biopsies?
I'm pretty sure I'm going to need one.

Julie, in an e-mail to
Mary Alderman, MD,
the morning after she discov-
ered a lump via breast self-
examination

Every breast cancer patient has her
own story to tell about the day she found her lump. Almost
to a woman, these stories share a common theme: a routine
or even mundane day indelibly marked by the unfamiliar
edges of a knot under the fingertips, a blurry but white-hot
image on an x-ray.

On June 25, 2009, I was in the shower, getting ready for a
gala event for my foundation, when my fingertips found my
lump. There had been something fibrous in this particular
location for years, and, during my monthly exam a couple of
weeks before, I'd made a mental note to check that it went back
down after my cycle. But now it was bigger, and the change
clearly hadn't happened in conjunction with my menstrual
cycle, which is when a woman can expect slight, hormon-
ally induced variations in the consistency of her breast tissue.
Something unusual was going on in my normally healthy
breasts; the pleasant sensation of warm water cascading over
my shoulders collided with the sickening sensation of just what
that something might be.

Breast cancer?

Anybody who tells you that their first reaction to the possibility of having cancer isn't to book a slow cruise up D'Nile River is either superhuman or telling a fib. Personally, my own denial was real, and lasted for about two seconds: years ago, when my daughter was showing the first unmistakable signs of autism, I had taken cover in denial for months, so I know first-hand how unproductive and frustrating that state of mind can be. I didn't want to live like that again.

I also know, as a physician, that beating cancer is a pro-active battle. I needed to know what this lump was, and if it turned out to be breast cancer, then I needed to go to war.

The key to surviving breast cancer is early detection.

Let me repeat that: *the key to surviving breast cancer is early detection.*

Screening—the process of testing for disease in a patient who is not displaying signs of that disease—is the key to early detection. That is because *there are no symptoms of early breast cancer*. Breast cancer begins in almost every case as a silent disease.

When I was a young girl, I liked to go on sleepovers with my girlfriends. We'd stay up late, trying out different kinds of make-up and talking about boys, and—almost invariably— ending up in the dark, a flashlight making the rounds, pointing upward and shining sinister light into the face of one girl or another as she told a ghost story, scaring each other silly. Thoroughly frightened out of our adolescent wits, we were then afraid to go to sleep, convinced that a ghost or a zombie or an escaped lunatic-convict-madman would creep silently into the suburban bedroom where we were slumbering and get us all. Our trick was to sneak down to the kitchen of the host's house and cart up armloads of her mother's pots and pans and place them just inside the bedroom door so, when that intruder tried to enter the room, the cookware would clatter noisily, waking us, alerting us to danger, calling in the experts—in this case, Mom and Dad—who would protect us from further harm. In the case of cancer, the silent cancer cells are the creeping intruder, and screening tools are the pots and pans that alert us to danger so we can call in the experts.

Screening and Diagnostic Tools

Breast Self-Examination (BSE)

The received wisdom used to be that regular breast self-examination (BSE) was among the finest screening tools, critical to early detection, and that it should be as routine a monthly habit as brushing your teeth is a daily one. Up until quite recently, every woman was encouraged—indeed, *exhorted*—to perform a BSE every twenty-eight days or so, with the optimal time to do it being right after her period ends.

HOW TO PERFORM A MONTHLY BREAST SELF-EXAMINATION (BSE)

THERE ARE FIVE STEPS IN A PROPERLY PERFORMED STANDARD BSE.

1. Stand in front of a mirror. Observe your breasts, first with your arms at your sides, second with them raised high over your head and, finally, with your hands pressing firmly on your hips to flex your chest muscles. Your breasts will likely be slightly different from each other—few women have completely symmetrical breasts—and this should not be a cause for concern. What you are looking for are these warning signs of cancer: a change in the shape or size of the breasts; any puckering or dimpling of the skin; swelling, redness or darkening of the breast; a rash or a scaly or crusty sore around the nipple area. Ask yourself a few questions to assess other warning signs: Have you experienced a pulling sensation in your nipple or other area of your breast? An unexplained feeling of warmth? Itchiness around the nipple? A new, unexplained pain in one particular spot that won't go away? A sudden or un-explained discharge from the nipple?

2. When you are taking a shower, with your left arm behind your head, use your right hand to examine your left breast. With flat fingers, using firm but gentle pressure, press down toward your chest wall on your breast in a spiraling mo-

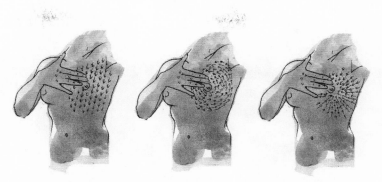

In a proper self breast examination, you can use your fingers to work either outward from the nipple, or inward toward the nipple, but the point is to cover the entire breast area, checking for any lumps or thickening in the breast tissue.

There is a big *however* at this juncture. Some studies support BSE as an effective screening tool, and others do not. Two major studies, one conducted in China and one in Russia and involving over a quarter a million women, concluded that there was no difference in breast cancer mortality rates after a fifteen-year period between those women who regularly performed BSEs and those who didn't.[37] Further, the same study found that, among the group of women who did perform regular BSEs, there were many more *false positives*—test results that indicate a person has a disease when, in fact, she does not. These false positives led to nearly twice as many breast biopsies with benign outcomes as resulted among the women in the group that did not perform BSEs.[38]

37 J.P Kösters, P.C. Gøtzsche, "Regular self-examination or clinical examination for early detection of breast cancer" (review). Cochrane Database Syst Rev. Issue 3: CD003373, 2008.

38 Ibid.

tion. You can work either outward from the nipple, or inward toward the nipple, but the point is to cover the entire breast area, checking for any lumps or thickening in the breast tissue. When you are done examining your left breast, switch sides and repeat the examination on your right. Before you get out of the shower, be sure to examine the axilla as described below.

3. A monthly breast self-exam should include examination of the armpit, or axilla, where all of the lymph nodes that drain the breast are located. The axilla is not a hollow or a flat surface as we think of it when we are putting on deodorant or shaving. Because the armpit isn't really flat, it's more complicated to examine than just running your fingers over it like we do a razor or wash-cloth. Think about this for a minute—your armpit is a pyramid. Seriously. Visualize the pyramids in Egypt, shrink one down in your mind's eye so it would fit in the palm of your hand, and then imagine fitting it, apex (top) first, in your armpit. It would fit because your axilla has an apex and four sides, just like a pyramid. And you need to examine all the sides well to do a complete axillary exam. Let's identify the top and the sides of the pyramid. The apex, or top of the pyramid, is deep inside our bodies at the rib cage and there are four walls—or the base of the pyramid—projecting from this apex. The anterior, or front wall of the pyramid, is formed by the pectoralis or chest wall muscle. The posterior, or back wall of the pyramid, is formed by the latissimus muscle, the one that gives a weight lifter

the look of a broad back. The outside or lateral wall of the pyramid is formed by the arm itself, and the inner or medial wall of the pyramid is formed by the chest wall. When examining the left axilla, place your left hand on your left hip, and use the fingers of your right hand to feel along all four of these walls of the pyramid, looking for any lumps. Be sure to reach as deeply as you can into your armpit, trying to feel all the way to the apex of that pyramid. After you finish the left side, examine the right side with your left hand.

4. The second phase of the examination of the left axilla involves placing your left hand on your head. This changes the shape of your armpit's pyramid, so that the front and back walls all but disappear, and making it much easier to get at that apex. Feel the inside and outside walls carefully for lumps, and be sure to feel as deeply as you can, reaching all the way to the apex on both sides of your body.

5. After you get out of the shower, lie down on your bed. Put a pillow under your left shoulder and your left arm behind your head. In this position, use the right hand to repeat on your left breast the firm, gentle, circular examination you preformed in the shower, checking carefully for any knots, lumps and thickenings. When you are done examining your left breast, switch sides and repeat the examination on your right. The final step of the breast exam is to sit up and gently squeeze each nipple, checking for discharge.

This is rather stark evidence that monthly breast self-examinations aren't truly the shiny, golden key to early detection that the medical community once promoted them to be. Indeed, such venerable organizations as the American Cancer Society now consider BSE an optional breast cancer screening tool.[39]

The reality is that no screening tool is 100% accurate. Mammography is widely believed to be such a precise technology, able to detect every cell of every breast cancer, that it is nearly magical. While such an enchanted tool would be most welcome, we all know that *magic* best belongs in the portfolios of fantasy writers and performers like Penn & Teller. The reality is that mammograms miss up to 20% of breast cancers.[40]

On the other hand, some statistics indicate that up to 40% of breast cancers are detected by the patient herself during the course of breast self-examination.[41] Anecdotally, I discovered my *own* breast cancer during a routine BSE. For both statistical and personal reasons, then, I think it is less than wise to discount BSE as a valuable, life-saving screening tool.

Further, I suggest that there are two ways in which breast self-examination can become an even more effective method for detecting breast cancer. First is practicing the proper technique. Giving oneself a thorough and competent BSE is a

---

39 http://www.cancer.org/acs/groups/content/@illinois/documents/document/octoberpresentation1pdf.pdf.

40 http://www.cancer.gov/cancertopics/factsheet/detection/mammograms.

41 *http://www.nationalbreastcancer.org/breast-self-exam*

quick, painless, and simple process, but—like anything that is simple; cooking up a hard-boiled egg to perfection, say, so that the yolk isn't coated with that telltale greenish layer that gives away the impatience of the cook—the nuances in how it is done are everything.

Second, I'd like to propose that the real basis of breast health is a woman's life-long knowledge of what her own healthy breast tissue feels like. There must be a foundation—a baseline—for monitoring breast health, and for comparing changes that might occur in the breast over the course of a lifetime. In order to perform a BSE effectively, a woman needs to know what it is that her fingertips are searching for.

As noted in the previous chapter, what we commonly refer to as "lumps" are really the differences between the feel of the breast lobes in relation to the breast fat—and lobes are, by their nature, "lumpy." How is someone supposed to tell the difference between the naturally bumpy topography of breast structure and what is an abnormal protuberance unless she has an intimate understanding of what her own healthy breast feels like?

Simply put: a breast is not a breast is not a breast. What are normal variations in the feel or consistency of one breast for one woman may be warning signs for another; and what feels perfectly ordinary in one part of one breast may be a warning sign if felt in another part of the same breast. That is, the tissues in various parts of the breast can feel different. The area under the armpit, for example, tends to have the most discernable natural "lumps." The areas under the breast, under the nipple, and toward the collarbone can all have their unique textures as well: the area under your breast might naturally feel like grains of rice, while the area under mine feels sandy; your nipple may feel as if it rests over a bed of pebbles while mine feels like lumpy mashed potatoes. In order to know what is a warning sign for her unique breasts, a woman first has to become intimately familiar with her singular topography.

When is the best time to start becoming familiar with one's own breast structure? When the breasts are healthy. Unless a woman is aware of the look as well as the feel of her own healthy breasts, it is difficult to make the comparison with what may be disease—to accurately assess when something has gone awry. Look at it this way: cookbooks often come with pictures of how a dish is optimally supposed to look when it is fully cooked and ready for presentation at the dinner table. This is what we are aiming for: knowledge of what our own breasts look and feel like at their optimum health so that, when and if there is a change in that level of health, it is readily detectible. So pick a day—a few days after your period ends, when your breasts are least tender or, for postmenopausal women, an easy day to remember, like the first of the month—and make a most important date with yourself.

When is the best time to begin gaining this knowledge? I say at puberty.

Many mothers, our own mothers and even ourselves often included, can be so absorbed by the "sex talk" that is our duty to our pubescent daughters, we forget that this talk is really not all about the sex *act* but the gender-related changes that are occurring in the young woman's body. Puberty, as we all know, is when hormones start to kick in and cause the beginning of breast development. It is at this early stage that young women need to be empowered to begin the good habit of breast self-examination. They should also, at this stage, be in possession of some very basic facts about their growing breasts so that they are not alarmed by the changes—and changing sensations—they are likely to see and feel as their breasts grow. Minimally, a young woman needs to know 1) that when she is young, she can expect her breast tissue to be fibrous and dense; 2) it is likely that at some point during the menstrual cycles her breasts will become tender, and generally "lumpier" than at other times of the month; 3) that this tenderness and lumpiness usually goes away when the cycle has, for that month, run its course. She should also know that breast cancer is so extremely rare in young women under twenty that it could be considered a "medical curiosity."[42] In *postpubertal* girls— meaning girls in the period following puberty—any lumps that are found turn out to be, in the vast majority of cases, benign conditions such as cysts, though we do recommend that such lumps be evaluated by a physician because there are rare cases in which breast cancer has been discovered in teenage girls. In *prepubertal* girls, or those who have yet to enter fully into puberty, the breast "bud" or disc—a one to two inch mass beneath the nipple that is getting ready to develop into a full-blown breast— can be mistaken for an ominous "lump" by

---

42 http://www.ncbi.nlm.nih.gov/pmc/articles/PMC1602749/?page=1.

concerned parents, presenting in some cases as asymmetrical breast development; removal of this disc would be disastrous, as the breast would then never develop.

The bottom line is that parents should be sensitive to the information that their own unique young girl needs and is able to process as her body changes, keeping in mind that the goal is to lay a foundation that fosters a life-long awareness of, and respect for, the importance of breast health. When adolescent girls are in my office for their yearly physicals, I regularly instruct them in self-breast examination, suggest that they put a monthly reminder on their cell phone calendars, and encourage them to remind mom to do hers as well every month when they are doing their own.

No matter at what age we finally get acquainted with our own breasts, however, general knowledge of breast structure, and of our own inimitable breast anatomy, can help us to take tender, loving, life-long care of our *girls*—and to distinguish between what are common, benign breast conditions and changes in our breasts that are cause for deeper concern.

Clinical Breast Examination (CBE)

A clinical breast examination is a breast exam that is done by a health professional—a doctor, a nurse practitioner, or other medical staff. It is part of the annual breast cancer screening that all women should begin having on or right after their twentieth birthday. Often, but not always, a CBE is a standard part of an annual physical examination. Before we talk specifically about the CBE, however, let me take a few paragraphs to talk about the importance of the old-fashioned annual physical exam.

There is a bit of a debate these days about the necessity for these annual exams.[43] Some doctors argue that the risks associated with some screening tests, such as radiation associated with mammograms, and the costs to the health care system, by some estimates as much as $350 million a year,[44] are exorbitant relative to the benefits. The majority of physicians, however, Ankit and myself included, continue to believe that the annual physical should be considered a standard part of a holistic, wellness-oriented approach to life.[45] Some examples of important, annual and age-specific tests include blood pressure readings, urine analysis screens for diabetes and kidney problems, and fecal occult blood tests to check for colorectal cancer—all of these are or should be part of a comprehensive annual exam as they aid doctor and patient in the early detection of disease. And early detection and prompt treatment are not only the keys to *surviving* disease but to *reversing damage* caused by disease. For example, a patient who, during her annual physical exam, discovers that her blood work shows elevated cholesterol levels that weren't present just the year before—say, a level over 200 mg/dl—will likely be advised by her doctor that a more

43 *http://www.ncbi.nlm.nih.gov/pubmed/17602927.*

44 http://health.usnews.com/health-news/articles/2007/09/24/do-you-actually-need-a-physical-exam.

45 http://archinte.ama-assn.org/cgi/content/short/165/12/1347.

detailed evaluation of her LDL (the "bad" cholesterol), HDL (the "good" cholesterol), triglyceride blood levels ("fatty acids," in the most basic sense), and perhaps a "Berkeley" test to see what her body is actually doing with the cholesterol is required. This is because, over time, if our bodies poorly handle cholesterol, arteries may narrow, resulting in poor blood flow not only to the heart but to the brain and other organs that, in turn, could result in strokes and heart attacks. By discovering early that she has an elevated cholesterol level, a person can take steps, such as changing her diet, exercising vigorously, and losing weight, that bring the levels back down within healthier parameters, and thus not only stop on-going damage and narrowing to her arteries but reverse any damage that another year of living with the higher levels might have caused. You know the old saying, "A stitch in time saves nine?" It means, of course, that when you notice a tiny hole in the seam of your blouse, if you sew it up right away it won't get worse. Same thing holds for your arteries: the sooner you address the problem, the sooner you can repair the damage and keep it from getting worse.

The most important part of your annual physical exam, however, isn't actually the medical tests themselves that your doctor will perform or order to be performed. The most important part of the exam is the time you and your doctor spend talking together, reviewing your medical history, your family's medical history, and the lifestyle choices you make and how they impact your health. Do you drink alcohol? How much? How often? Do you smoke? Are you exposed on a regular basis to second-hand smoke? How often do you exercise? What kind of exercise do you perform? Does this include regular cardio-vascular workouts? What is your typical daily diet? Have you gained weight over the course of the year since your last visit? Lost weight? How much? Why? What supplements do you take? What medications, both over-the-counter and prescription meds do you take? How many hours of sleep do you get, on average, each night? Do you sleep through the night or do you wake often, or struggle with insomnia? Do you *work* overnight? Questions such as these can help your doctor to probe more deeply, discover habits or conditions in your life that may expose you to health risks and, so, be able to assess and recommend preventative measures to cancel or mitigate the risks.

We'll talk in more depth about risks associated specifically with breast cancer later in this book, but as an immediate example, did you know that working overnight—as, for instance, nurses on night shift do—can increase your risk for developing breast cancer?[46] Researchers believe that this has something to do with the production of melatonin, a naturally occurring compound related to regulation of circadian rhythms and sleep patterns whose production is powerfully stimulated by cycles of light and dark—cycles that are profoundly disrupted for those who regularly clock in on the graveyard shift. A once-a-year appointment with your doctor can help you to focus year-round on your physical well being,

---

46 http://jnci.oxfordjournals.org/content/93/20/1563.full.

alert you to the choices and changes you can make to enhance your overall health—and so *prevent* disease altogether.

But let's not kid ourselves: this kind of comprehensive, talk-intensive sort of annual physical is, indeed, old-fashioned. One can blame this on a modern, overburdened health system in which the number of caseloads most doctors carry doesn't afford them the luxury of quality time with each patient, or on an insurance system that promotes disease treatment rather than disease prevention by virtue of the simple fact that annual, preventative physical examinations are often not covered by health insurance premiums. If you want holistic, wellness care these days, you will likely need to spend time searching out a specialized physician who will supply it, and likely have to pay an out-of-pocket premium for the service. Whatever one blames the problem on, however, the solution is not to ignore the problem—it is instead to find a way to ensure that you take care of yourself annually and properly, even if it's an out-of-pocket cost. This personal gift, in the longer term, both saves lives and lowers the exorbitant costs of treating disease that might have been prevented.

In any case, a CBE should be a standard part of every woman's annual physical examination, or, if a full physical is not part of an individual's routine, at the very least it should be a part of every woman's annual breast cancer screening. You will be asked to disrobe from the waist up and don one of those pretty paper robes that are so fashionable in the immediate environs of doctors' offices. Your doctor will first examine your breasts visually. She is looking for changes in breast size and changes in the skin on and surrounding your breasts, as well as signs of injury or infection. She may ask you to change the position of your arms during this phase of the examination—lift them over your head, or lean forward and press your palms together to tighten the muscles beneath the breasts—to better evaluate their physical presentation.

Next, your doctor will ask you to lie flat on the examining table so that she can palpate each breast individually. If she is examining your left breast, she will ask you to place your left hand behind your head and, if it is the right breast, the right hand. She will gently press on the breast from about one inch below the breast, all the way up to the collarbone, in the armpit, and along the neck, checking the breast tissue for "lumps" that are harder, larger, or in any way substantially different from the way that your general breast tissue feels, as well as for swollen lymph nodes. She will also gently squeeze your nipple, checking for any discharge. This is, not incidentally, the absolute prime time for a patient, if she is at all concerned about her own technique for breast self-examination, to ask for a refresher course in how to perform a BSE.

Except when your breasts are tender, the CBE is painless, and the risk factors to this screening procedure are nonexistent, save for the occasional false positive—those instances when a doctor sees or feels a change in the breast tissue for which she recommends further testing but which turns out not to have warranted concern. The downside of a false positive is that it can cause stress and worry in the interim between the CBE and follow-up testing, but in this case the negative of the stress is far outweighed by the possibility that the doctors recommendation may, indeed, be a life-saving intervention.

Mammography

Mammograms are, in essence, breast x-rays. They are the most reliable screening tool for breast cancer that we have today, detecting cancers that show up as a dense mass as well as microcalcifications, but detecting them when they are too small to be felt by a woman performing a BSE, or even a clinician performing a CBE—finding them before they have a chance to grow, when they are still most responsive to treatment.

When to get a mammogram is a matter of some debate. Every year? Every two years? At what age? The United States Preventative Services Task Force recommended biennial screenings only for women who are between the ages of fifty and seventy-four.[47] This recommendation came under fire as grossly under-screening women when it was released in 2010. For women who are at average risk for breast cancer, most institutions, including the American Cancer Society, Komen, Planned Parenthood, and the National Cancer Institute recommend a mammogram every year after a woman turns forty,[48]

---

47 http://www.uspreventiveservicestaskforce.org/uspstf/uspsbrca.htm.

48 *http://www.cancer.org/healthy/findcancerearly/cancerscreeningguidelines/ american-cancer-society-guidelines-for-the-early-detection-of-cancer; http://*

DCIS

CHANGING DIAGNOSTIC AND TREATMENT STANDARDS?

DCIS stands for *Ductal Carcinoma In Situ*, a very early stage or pre-cancer that has not spread outside of the breast's milk ducts; indeed, *in situ* is Latin for "in its original place." There has lately been some confusion around a diagnosis of DCIS, with some scientists referring to it as a cancer that has not spread and others who believe it should not be called a cancer at all. But this is more than a language problem, of course, because what you call it helps determine how you and your doctor decide to treat it.

In order to put the current debate about treatment of DCIS into perspective, we need to begin with the understanding that breast cancer is really a spectrum of diseases that start with pre-cancer and non-invasive cancer, and extend to invasive cancer and metastatic cancer; the definition and treatment for each is both fluid (changing and improving as researchers discover new treatments and protocols) and custom (each woman's cancer is different, as are her reasons for choosing one treatment option over another). There is no means to accurately predict if any single DCIS will spread and become life threatening or if it won't. The best indication we have at this time is that approximately half of all DCISs will become invasive cancer within twenty to thirty years of their appearance. The EBM (Evidence-Based Medicine) guidelines currently recommend a conservative approach to treatment and, until more clinical trials are completed and the medical community has more hard evidence in hand that suggests a change in treatment is warranted, we concur.

with a CBE at least every three years after the age of twenty. As already discussed, I believe that an annual mammogram, beginning the year that a woman turns forty, is probably optimal for women who are at average risk for the disease.

The reason some doctors or organizations may give for backing off their recommendations for more frequent use of mammograms as a screening tool is the radiation that they, like every other x-ray, involve. While it is always a good idea to avoid exposure to excess radiation when possible, the amount a woman receives during a normal mammogram is very low, about 70 millirems—or about the same dose each of us receives from exposure to our everyday environment over a period of two to three months, and special care is taken to use the lowest dose possible and still provide an accurate mammographic image. Moreover, radiation facilities are monitored by national and international protection agencies, and modern x-ray machines have tightly controlled, filtrated beams that prevent the radiation from scattering to other parts of the patient's body, where the beam has not been specifically directed. A woman should never undergo any kind of an x-ray while she is pregnant, but in most every other case, the life-saving benefits of having a mammogram trump the exposure to a small dose of radiation every time.

That said, due to radiation exposure, only in special cases would I suggest a woman begin mammographic screening earlier than age thirty. A "special case" would, certainly, be when a woman has tested positive for BRCA1 or BRCA2. We'll talk in more depth about the BRCA genes later in this book but, for now, BRCA1 and BRCA2 are human genes that belong to a class of genes known as tumor suppressors, and mutation of these genes have been linked to not only hereditary breast cancer but hereditary ovarian cancer. In cases where a woman has tested positive for these genes, I would consider, at a minimum, annual mammograms starting when the woman reaches the age when she is *ten years younger* than her mother or other first-degree relative was at the time she was diagnosed. That is, as a general rule, if Mom was diagnosed with breast cancer at 42, her daughter should begin her annual mammograms at age 32. She might also want to consider an annual MRI, alternating the two screening tests every six months. In these cases where the genetic predisposition has been confirmed, undergoing prophylactic mastectomies is, of course, also an option, and one that is likely to become more and more common as women are inspired by public figures like Angelina Jolie. As Betty Ford and others like her, back in the day, changed the game and made it safe and acceptable for women to talk openly about the subject of breast cancer, so Ms. Jolie has started the important public conversation about prophylactic mastectomies.

Mammograms are, these days, fairly easily accessed. They're performed in radiology and imaging centers, hospital radiology departments, special mobile mammography vans and even some physicians' offices. They are also performed in specialty mammography clinics and breast health centers. While there is no possible way to make a generalized recommendation about which facility is best—taking into account the modernity of the equipment and the skill of the radiologists at every local mammography service—I tend to prefer mammography vans, or specialty mammography clinics and breast health centers for my mammograms, simply because this *is* their specialty. It is what they do every day; their personnel are usually well trained and their sensitivity to the anxieties of women who are undergoing the procedure is well honed.

One should not underestimate the value of sensitivity in a mammography setting. Setting aside for a moment the sober fact that some women are undergoing mammography as a further test to confirm a breast cancer diagnosis, the process can be anxiety-provoking even in women who are there simply out of routine. Let's just say it: painless as mammography really, truly is, none of us particularly relishes the idea of having her ta-tas squished.

The reality, of course, is that having a mammogram is usually pretty quickly done—the whole process takes about fifteen to twenty minutes—and mild discomfort is normally at the extreme end of physical response. To make the mammography go even more quickly, remember that you'll be undressing for the test from the waist up, so wear a shirt that you can take off easily, and avoid wearing deodorant or antiperspirant, perfumes or powders that you'll have to wash off, as certain ingredients common in these sort of products can show up on the resulting x-rays and make the results more difficult to interpret. If your breasts are particularly sensitive, taking an Advil or a Tylenol about an hour prior to the test can help reduce discomfort; if you are particularly anxious about the mammogram, let your technologist know as she can help guide you through the process in a way that reduces and alleviates your concerns.

The procedure itself will involve attaching a tiny metal ball to each nipple with special, non-pull adhesive tape. These balls will show up on the resulting x-rays and act as markers for the radiologist who is interpreting the results of your test. Then each breast is pressed between two plates, twice—once with the beam aimed from top to bottom, and once with the beam aimed from side to side. And that's all there is to it.

One final decision that a woman has to make about her mammography is whether to have a standard, or film mammography, or a digital one. The difference is that with a standard mammography, the x-ray images are captured on film, and with the digital sort the images are captured directly onto a computer. Less radiation is needed for digital mammography, and digital images can be more easily manipulated—lightened or darkened or enlarged, for example—so there is some benefit to the radiologist who is interpreting the results. Digital mammography results can also be more easily stored and shared electronically with other health care professionals. Additionally, for certain women—those who are under the age of fifty, either premenopausal or perimenopausal, or those whose breast tissue is naturally dense—digital mammography may be more accurate at detecting cancer. Not all facilities are equipped with digital equipment, however, and not all insurance plans cover the additional cost, so if you or your doctor prefer digital mammography, make sure you check with both the facility where your test is to be performed and your insurance carrier prior to having the procedure.

Mammograms, as I've said, are often the first screening tests performed after a woman has discovered a lump, either by way of a BSE or a CBE, to rule out a suspicion of breast cancer or as a further step in the diagnostic process. Ideally, however, they are used as an annual, routine screening tool to promote wellness and peace of mind. The percentage of women who actually avail themselves of this important tool, however, is no where near as high as most doctors would like to see it—hovering at between 66 to 68% for white, black and Asian women, and dropping to only 61% for Latinas.[49] The excuse I hear most often among my patients who neglect this basic health procedure is that they simply forget to do it—even when I supply them with a lab order! Many doctors, however, are taking a unique but simple step to do away with this particular excuse—they are sending annual reminder letters to their patients. In a study conducted by researchers at the San Diego State University Graduate School of Public Health, women who received an annual reminder letter from either their doctor or a mammography facility were over twice as likely to actually have the test as those who did not receive a letter.[50] We recommend you work with a doctor or breast health center that has implemented such a reminder system.

---

49 http://www.cdc.gov/cancer/breast/statistics/screening.htm.

50 http://www.ncbi.nlm.nih.gov/pubmed/11006056.

Breast Ultrasound

Ultrasound, or medical sonography, is an imaging technology that uses sound waves to capture the images of many internal organs as well as muscles and tendons, in real time. Most of us are familiar with obstetric ultrasound, those wondrous images of our children in utero, but ultrasound is also used as a diagnostic tool for many other conditions, including cardiac, renal (kidney), liver and eye problems. It is also used in the detection of breast cancer and other breast conditions.

An ultrasound is a noninvasive medical procedure that is completely painless—in fact, the worst I have personally heard from any woman who has experienced one is that it can be a bit ticklish and a little sloppy. A clear, or sometimes green- or blue-colored gel, that has usually been gently warmed, is first applied to the breast or other part of the body to be imaged, and then a transducer—a device that sends and receives sound waves—is placed on top of the gel. The gel is a conductive medium that helps the sound waves pass into a person's body where they then "bounce" off the organ or tissue, creating a picture for the doctor to view.

Often an ultrasound is the first test a clinician will order when the results of a mammogram are suspicious, because ultrasound images are able to show all areas of the breast, including the areas closest to the wall of the chest that are difficult to capture in a mammogram. With the use of ultrasound, your doctor can tell if the lump he felt is a mass, or if it is filled with fluid (a cyst), and then, because of the real time nature of ultrasound images, he can use the technology to guide in the placement of the fine needle used to aspirate a cyst or to collect a biopsy sample from a mass. Further, some ultrasound machines have Doppler capabilities, a special ultrasound technique that allows whoever is performing the sonogram—a doctor or technician—to see the blood flow in veins and arteries. In the case of breast tissue, the doctor will be able to evaluate the blood flow, or lack of blood flow, to a breast mass, providing him with further information that may help to determine its cause.

With ultrasound images, your doctor can also monitor the size of a benign but persistent cyst, more readily locate the cause of other benign breast complaints such as pain or swelling. And, more importantly for women who have been diagnosed with cancer, ultrasound can help to determine whether or not the cancer has spread to the axillary lymph nodes in the armpits.

Because sonography uses sound waves to create its resulting images—that is, there is no potentially harmful radiation involved in ultrasound—there has been some interest in the technology as a substitute for mammograms. The problem with such substitution is that breast ultrasound testing finds too many details to be a good general screening tool. If we used ultrasound for routine screening, there would be a tremendous number of unnecessary second studies to clarify all of the minute details sonography found, and/or a lot of unnecessary biopsies. Sonography appears to have a great role to play in the health care of women with dense breast tissue, or with silicone breast implants. In those situations, sonograms can show good pictures of targeted areas in much greater detail than mammography can. However, except for those specific targeted areas of interest, we recommend sticking to the mammogram as the primary screening tool of choice.

Thermography

Thermography, or Digital Infrared Imaging, uses heat, or body temperature, as a diagnostic tool. The principle behind the technology is that the blood flow as well as the metabolic activity is, in almost all cases, higher in tissue that is pre-cancerous or that surrounds a breast cancer. This is because, in order to constantly feed themselves—attract nutrients that are carried through the blood—cancer cells cause existing blood vessels to stay open, open dormant ones, and even cause new blood vessels to be created by the body. All of this vascular activity, in turn, increases the surface temperature of the skin and other tissues that surround the cancer. The process of thermography creates a map of the resulting heat, a unique infrared image of the breast that, some studies indicate, may be a useful tool in interpreting high risk for breast cancer.[51]

Thermography is exquisitely sensitive, able to detect metabolic changes at their earliest stages, in their smallest presence, and it does so by using infrared light—that is, without

---

[51] http://www.iact-org.org/patients/breastthermography/what-is-breast-therm.html.

radiation and the potential harm it can cause. Well, then! Why hasn't thermography replaced mammography? Because there is a big *however* waiting around this corner, too: thermography, because it looks at heat, has a tremendous number of variables that must be controlled in order for the exams to be reliable. For example, from year to year to year, the room temperature, the technician and camera and, much more difficult to control, the patient's metabolism needs to be consistent. When we consider that women being screened for breast cancer are of child-bearing age and their weight, thyroid function and metabolism may undergo significant shifts, interpreting thermography can be a tremendous challenge. The value of thermography, its accuracy, is completely dependent on both controlling the myriad variables very tightly and the length of time that it is consistently used. Still, I see potential for thermography as a diagnostic tool in very specific—and long-term—settings. Let me explain.

The thermographic map I mentioned above is, in fact, unique to every person; every person's personal map is utterly one-of-a-kind. What might qualify as an area of concern on my map may be a perfectly ordinary biological norm for you. The trick to finding out what is normal for each individual depends on being able to compare the map from year to year to year and observe the changes in the map. In order to use thermography to efficiently and accurately detect cancers, one must first find a thermography facility and a technician that she likes and is willing to work with over the long haul—and I am talking a lifetime here—and begin with a "baseline" heat map. The next year—at the same time of the month, at the same facility and with the same technician doing the procedure, and the same team interpreting the results—do another map. Then *compare* the maps—and then compare them again with the map that is taken the next year and the year after that and ten years from now, because it is not the map itself but the *changes* in the map that indicate areas of concern. As a one-time snapshot of breast health, thermography is not practical or useful; as a lifetime tool that is rigorous in terms of constancy, yes, it has the potential to be a screening tool for certain individuals who are dedicated and consistent in pursuing their health.

MRI (Magnetic Resonance Imaging)

Magnetic Resonance Imaging is a powerful diagnostic tool that can provide doctors and patients with information obtainable in no other way. After a CBE, a mammogram and/or an ultrasound, for example, has been done, and still more information is needed to make an accurate diagnosis of breast cancer—or, when a doctor detects a mass during a CBE but the mass is not showing up on mammograms or with ultrasounds—MRI can be brought into play to clarify the diagnosis. The technology can also be used to fine-tune a course of cancer treatment as it allows doctors to see the size of a diagnosed cancer, if the cancer involves the muscle that underlies the breast, and if lymph nodes have enlarged significantly, indicating that a cancer has spread. During cancer treatment, if chemotherapy is one of the cancer-fighting tools that are being deployed, and if the chemo is being administered prior to surgery, MRI is often used to monitor how the chemo is working, if and by how much the tumor is shrinking. In cases of recurring cancer, when a woman has previously undergone a lumpectomy, it can be the imaging tool of choice as mammograms often cannot tell the difference between what is scar tissue and what is a new cancer mass. For women who opt for post-mastectomy breast implants, MRI is simply the best way to tell if a silicone implant has ruptured. And, though not a substitute for a mammogram, as mammograms can detect some cancers that even the potent MRI cannot, it can be used as a routine screening tool when a woman has a very high risk of breast cancer based on such factors as family history.

MRI works by creating a magnetic field around, and directing radio waves at your body to produce detailed, 3-D images. There is no radiation involved in the MRI process and no discomfort, as the body cannot feel radio waves. But there are still some risks that patients need to be aware of. As with other imaging technologies, there is the possibility of a false positive diagnosis, in this case particularly for premenopausal women, as hormone fluctuations that happen during the menstrual cycle can make the test results more difficult to interpret. Studies have found that the optimum time to schedule an MRI for women who still have their periods is during the *follicular phase*, or between days three and fourteen of a normal twenty-eight-day cycle.[52] Understandably then, scheduling an MRI for a woman with an irregular cycle becomes, while not impossible, problematic. Additionally, we note that MRIs are generally avoided for pregnant women, and that a woman who is breastfeeding should be prepared to stop for at least two days after the procedure in order for the dyes that are frequently, though not always, administered intravenously in conjunction with the procedure to have a chance to flush out of her system. It is these dyes that are a primary concern when considering risks associated with MRI. Used in order to make the images more distinct and easier for your doctor to interpret, the dyes can cause allergic reactions and have also been known to cause serious problems in women who have kidney problems.

The procedure itself, excepting the pinprick that accompanies the insertion of the IV line, is painless and noninvasive. You'll be asked to change into a gown, and to remove jewelry and other metals that can damage the machinery during the procedure. You'll also need to tell your doctor about any implanted medical devices, including tissue expanders, pacemakers, a drug port or an artificial joint.

Then you'll lie face down on the scanning table, which is padded for your comfort, with your breasts resting in the table's hollow depressions. These depressions contain coils that will detect the machine's magnetic signals. You'll be given a microphone with which to communicate with the technician, who will be in a separate room during the process, and the

---

52 http://www.medscape.com/viewarticle/715815.

scanning table will then slide into the large, central opening of the MRI machine. It is at this point, when a patient is in the machine itself—in what can, indeed, feel like the smallish inside of a sterile tube, that a patient can begin to feel anxious, the uneasy feeling heightened because often the machine produces loud thumping or tapping sounds. Because the patient must lie quite still during the entire procedure, and the procedure can take up to an hour to complete, we recommend taking steps to address the potential for any discomfort beforehand. If you are at all claustrophobic, let the technician know; he or she can arrange for you to be given a mild sedative prior to the procedure. Ask for earplugs to muffle the noise inside the machine. Test out the microphone to reassure yourself that it is working and you have a ready means of communication with the world outside of the tube. Prepare yourself mentally; decide that you will use the time to meditate, or even to take a nap!

New Frontiers in Screening

Digital Tomosynthesis—newly approved by FDA and becoming ever more widely used—takes information gathered by x-ray and uses computer software to assemble images. The machine operates much like a panograph x-ray that dentists use, with an x-ray machine arm that moves in an arc over the breast while you stand still. The computer then uses the data set that was obtained with the single dose of radiation and assembles it in slices of variable thickness that are then interpreted by the radiologist. While Digital Tomosynthesis may be more sensitive, and more specific than other diagnostic radiation tools, it uses more radiation than standard mammography. What exactly its role will be in screening a population that is concerned about over-radiating women remains to be seen.

Another issue that is still being worked out is what additional training the technicians and physicians need to be able to optimize use of this screening tool. And, of course, the costs are always a consideration—insurers aren't reimbursing for it differently than mammography at this time, and yet it's a lot more work for physicians to interpret it. As a result, there may be an additional charge for digital tomosynthesis. As the issues get ironed out over the next several years, however, this new tool should be in wider use.

MBI (Molecular Breast Imaging)—this mode of imaging uses specialized gamma camera technology in combination with a nuclear medicine radiotracer called Technetium-99m that is injected intravenously. The tracer is "tagged" to a compound (called Sestamibi) that allows it to be taken up into the mitochondria, the energy powerhouses of the cell, an area that is much more active in cancer cells than in healthy cells. The tracer is detected by the specialized camera and can detect much smaller tumors than mammography can. The concern, however, remains the amount of radiation the tool requires. Radiation with MBI is about two to four times what a digital mammography exam entails, but MBI is more comfortable because it uses less compression than film screen mammography. Almost all of the radioactivity from the Technetium-99m leaves the body in about twenty-four hours, and Lumagen, a particular brand of MBI, has a special crystal in its camera allowing use of a lower dose of Technetium-99m. With its special camera and software, Lumagen uses about one-quarter the dose that is used in cardiac evaluations. MBI will likely have a role in screening dense breasts once the dose of radio-tracer is better established. Right now, MBI's role is probably in problem-solving when more imaging is needed to know if something that looks questionable on traditional imaging is hypermetabolic (as cancer is) or not (therefore less likely to be a cause for concern). The bonus in using MBI in this way is that it can save a woman an unnecessary biopsy; the minus is that it involves additional radiation, and also requires a radio-active agent to be injected into the body. Medicare is paying for the procedure as of this writing, and insurance is beginning to pay for it; it is less expensive than MRI, but it is more expen-sive than mammography.

Tissue Sampling and Biopsy

A breast biopsy is indisputably the best way to evaluate an abnormality in the breast and determine if it is cancer. A sam-ple of the tissue in the suspicious area is removed from the breast and sent to a lab where technicians can work directly with the cells that make up the lump or mass in the area of concern and identify any abnormalities.

There are a variety of ways in which your doctor can obtain a sample of tissue from your breast, and she's likely to choose one method or another based on the characteristics of your particular suspicious lump or mass: its location, its size, its texture, and so on. Some methods of tissue sampling are more invasive than others and, consequently, more or less uncomfortable or anxiety-provoking. Most every doctor you'll ever meet, however, will cite the easing of her patient's fears during this sensitive time as one of her primary concerns, so if you want to better understand why she chose a particular method of sampling in your case, just ask.

Fine-needle aspiration is the most uncomplicated way to remove sample tissue from the breast and is often used when your doctor discovers a lump during a CBE, in order to immediately distinguish between a lump that might be a fluid-filled cyst and one that is cause for greater concern and, subsequently, further testing. It is a quick and relatively painless procedure done by inserting a syringe equipped with an extremely fine needle into the lump and withdrawing a sample of cells or fluid. If no fluid can be withdrawn, or if the lump doesn't go away on its own, your doctor will most likely recommend further testing, such as a mammogram or an ultrasound.

A *core needle biopsy* is used most commonly to evaluate a lump or mass that your doctor can palpate in the course of a CBE and/or that can also be seen on a diagnostic image, such as a mammogram or ultrasound. A surgeon or a radiologist will use a thin needle to remove several tissue samples, each about the size of a grain of rice, from the suspicious area. Diagnostic imaging technologies, such as mammography, ultrasound and MRI, can be used for this procedure to guide your surgeon in correctly positioning the needle. The collected samples are then sent to a lab for analysis.

Stereotactic biopsy uses mammography technology to exactly pinpoint a suspicious lump or mass and is often employed when the abnormality is too small to be easily felt by hand. You will lie facedown on a special biopsy table that has holes through which a breast can be positioned. The table is padded for your comfort—especially nice as this procedure can take up to an hour to perform. The table is then raised several feet as the radiologist performs this procedure from beneath the table. The breast is pressed between two plates, just as it is during a routine mammogram, and images are taken that will guide the radiologist to the exact location he wants to biopsy. He will make a small incision, usually no more than half an inch long, and then use either a hollow needle or a vacuum-powered probe to remove several tissue samples to send to a lab to be analyzed. Similarly, *ultrasound-guided core needle biopsy* and *MRI-guided core needle biopsy* use those imaging technologies to guide the radiologist to the exact location of the suspicious lump or mass.

A *surgical biopsy* is most commonly performed in a hospital operating room, on an out-patient basis, with the use of both sedation and a local anesthetic. There are two types of surgical biopsy: an *incisional biopsy*, during which a portion of the suspicious mass is removed so that it can be sent to a lab for analysis, and *excisional biopsy*, also called a lumpectomy, during which the entire suspicious mass as well as a small margin of normal tissue are removed. The difference between the two, in general, is that an incisional biopsy is performed for diagnostic purposes, and a lumpectomy, followed by a course of radiation therapy, is currently the standard treatment procedure for early breast cancers involving a mass of less than an inch diameter.

Sometimes a technique called *wire localization* will be used during surgical biopsy, especially in cases where the breast mass cannot be readily palpated. This entails the insertion of a thin wire into the breast mass prior to surgery; your surgeon then uses this wire as a guide while he is operating. He may also, during the course of the biopsy, insert a minuscule steel clip inside your breast at the biopsy site; this clip is then used as a marker to aid in monitoring the cancer site or in the event that further surgery must be performed at the same site.

Before undergoing any sort of breast biopsy, you likely will want to arrange to take the rest of the day off to take it easy. There could be soreness at the site of the biopsy, and you will be wrapped up tightly in big ace bandages after the procedure to compress the biopsy site and minimize swelling and bruising; ice packs, non-aspirin pain relievers such as Tylenol, a cozy chair and a hot cup of tea will be your best friends. After a surgical biopsy, you will more than likely have super glue closing your incision or perhaps stitches to care for as well.

It will, almost invariably, take several days before you and your doctor receive all the results of a core needle or a surgical biopsy from the lab. Different techniques of analysis require different lengths of time to accomplish, so the report may actually arrive over the course of several days, in the form of two or three separate reports. This or these reports—called your pathology report—will contain a great many details about your tissue samples, such as size and color and consistency of the tissue, as well as whether or not cancer cells were present.

We'll go into greater detail about what to look for in your pathology reports later in this book. For now, the central information you are looking for in a report prepared following a lumpectomy for breast cancer is whether or not the *margins*—the normal tissue surrounding the mass that was also removed during the procedure—are positive or negative. If they are positive, that means that cancer cells were found in the surrounding normal tissue, and your doctor will likely recommend further surgery to remove more tissue. If they are negative, or *clean*, it means that no cancer cells were found in the surrounding tissue and, in most cases, no additional surgery will be required at that time.

In the cases of core needle biopsies and incisional biopsies, the most important information you are looking for is whether or not the opinions of your radiologist and your pathologist are the same—and sometimes they are not. For example, the results of your MRI, performed by your radiologist, may suggest cancer, but your pathologist finds no cancer cells in your biopsy samples. In this case you will want to sit down with your doctor for a discussion about whether or not you need more testing and/or surgery to further evaluate.

If the pathology report clearly indicates that cancer is indeed present, well, then, it is on to the next step in the process of the cure.

Discovering a problem during

a breast cancer screening

does not always mean the

problem is breast cancer.

Ankit

Every day in my practice as a plastic surgeon specializing in breast reconstruction, I meet women who have been diagnosed with breast cancer and are exploring their surgical options. I also meet women who have a variety of other breast conditions—benign, but troublesome in other ways, causing physical or emotional discomfort. Familiarity with these conditions is important because they can be symptoms of breast cancer—or they can be mistaken for symptoms of breast cancer.

Common Benign Breast Conditions

Breast Pain

There are several reasons a woman might experience breast pain. Foremost among them is what is referred to as *cyclical breast pain*—the pain, or tenderness, that is a commonplace if frequently uncomfortable occurrence linked to the fibrocystic changes that happen during the menstrual cycle. These sort of fibrocystic changes refer to the range of completely normal changes within the breast tissue caused by cyclic shifts in the hormones estrogen and progesterone that cause the milk glands and ducts to enlarge and the breasts to swell and retain water. When the menstrual cycle is complete, the hormones once again settle down and the breasts return to their normal state. Similarly, pain associated with fibrocystic changes in breast tissue also occurs during menopause, when hormone levels are again shifting and the breasts are adjusting to new hormone norms. Treatments include over-the-counter pain relievers such as Advil or Motrin (ibuprofen), or Aleve (naproxen), or the prescription of oral contraceptives that lower the level of hormones that trigger the fibrocystic changes. It's important to note here that Julie feels very strongly about avoiding Tylenol (acetaminophen) as a pain reliever whenever possible because it decreases glutathione synthesis. Most of the time, if we need a pain reliever, something is wrong in the body and more, not less, glutathione, is needed. Sometimes a prescription drug called Danazol can be recommended for breast pain that is severe, but the caution here is that Danazol works by mimicking a male sex hormone and the side effects can include the growth of unwanted body hair as well as acne.

Non-cyclical breast pain is the overall term for pain that is not associated with the menstrual cycle. This type of pain can be caused by a blocked milk duct; *mastitis*, which is an infection of the breast tissue that most commonly occurs in women who are breast-feeding; *chondritis*, or an inflammation in the rib cage that can feel so intense it is often mistaken for a heart attack; a strained chest muscle; or a problem with the lung or blood circulation to the heart. Clearly, any breast pain that cannot be readily linked to the hormonal shifts of menstruation or menopause should be checked out by a physician, but it is important to note that breast pain is rarely a signal of breast cancer.

Fibrocystic Breasts

In the old days (not so very long ago!), this condition was referred to as fibrocystic breast *disease*, but since more than half of all women will experience some sort of fibrocystic breast changes in their lifetimes, it is now simply known as "having fibrocystic breasts." Fibrocystic breasts are characterized by "ropey" or thick-feeling, scar-like breast tissue, lumps that can result from enlarged breast lobules, fluctuation in the size of these lumps, and even a dark but non-bloody nipple discharge. The condition is experienced mostly by women in their premenopausal years, because, again, it is believed to be triggered by hormonal shifts and, so, it is only rarely experienced among postmenopausal women unless they are on hormone therapy. Having fibrocystic breasts does not increase a woman's risk of breast cancer, though if the fluctuations in the size, shape, or density of familiar lumps, bumps or ropes persist after the end of a menstrual period, or if a new lump appears, these developments should be evaluated by a doctor.

Fibroadenomas

Fibroadenomas are solid, smooth, often rubbery but sometimes hard tumors that have a distinct, well-defined shape, move easily beneath the skin when palpated and are generally fairly small. Ones that are hard can feel, in fact, as if there are marbles within the breast tissue, a sensation that can be disconcerting, but they are painless and non-cancerous. Fibroadenomas occur most often in adolescents and women under thirty. They are thought to be brought on by the influx of reproductive hormones that begins in puberty. Indeed, these tumors can grow in size during the hormonal shifts caused by pregnancy, and shrink in size as hormone production decreases during menopause. Though these tumors will sometimes simply disappear of their own accord, some women opt to have them surgically removed for either aesthetic reasons—they can alter the shape and feel of the breast—or for peace of mind. Fibroadenomas, again, are not cancerous though the careful caveat applies here, too: if changes in shape or texture are noted, they should be checked by a doctor to see if they are *complex fibroadenoma* that can contain calcifications and do slightly increase the risk of breast cancer.

Breast Cysts

Cysts are fluid-filled, roundish sacs that can feel, frankly, as if there is a grape, or sometimes many grapes, lodged beneath the skin of the breast. They are common in women in their later reproductive years, the 30s and 40s, and most often simply disappear with menopause unless, again, the woman is on hormone therapy. Most cysts require no treatment, as they do not increase a woman's risk of breast cancer, but if one is large or causes discomfort or pain, there are treatment options. A doctor can perform a procedure called fine-needle aspiration, in which a thin needle is inserted into the breast cyst and the fluid inside is removed (aspirated). If no fluid can be withdrawn, if the fluid contains blood, or if the lump that the cyst has caused does not resolve after aspiration, the doctor may opt for additional tests, such as sending the fluid to a laboratory for analysis, or mammography or ultrasound. The use of oral contraceptives for premenopausal women can help to reduce the recurrence of these cysts, as can the discontinuance of hormone therapy for postmenopausal women, as these cysts are thought to be stimulated by an excess of estrogen. In some cases—if the cyst or cysts are painful, if they recur frequently, or if analysis of the cyst fluid contains any troublesome signs— surgical removal is also an option.

Nipple Discharge

Any fluid that seeps from the nipple is referred to as nipple discharge, and even in women who aren't pregnant or breast-feeding, it isn't necessarily an abnormal event. The discharge may look white and cloudy, it may be yellow, green, brown or bloody, it may be thick and sticky or thin and watery, it may discharge spontaneously or it may discharge only when the nipple or breast is squeezed. The causes of nipple discharge are just as variable: fibroadenomas, hormone imbalance, breast infection, and even the use of some medications may be behind the problem. These are all benign conditions, but, importantly, breast cancer may also be a suspect, particularly if the woman experiencing the discharge is over forty years of age, if the discharge is accompanied by a palpable lump in the breast, if only one breast is affected, or if the discharge is bloody. In these cases, an evaluation by a physician is critical.

We'll talk more about male breast cancer later in this book, but it is essential to note here that men can also experience nipple discharge. In adolescent boys this is a fairly normal phenomenon as the hormone testosterone, as well as small amounts of estrogen, begin to stimulate the growth of secondary sex characteristics. In adult males, however, nipple discharge can be a cause for concern, and should in every case be evaluated by a physician.

Inverted Nipple

Inverted or *invaginated* nipple is a condition in which the nipple is retracted instead of protracting or pointing out of the breast. It can be congenital—meaning existing before birth or occurring in the first month of life—or caused by a variety of events including trauma to the breast that results in scar tissue, sagging breasts, and tuberculosis. Often thought of as a wholly aesthetic issue, this condition has implications for breastfeeding women, who can find the process more difficult and/or painful than women with normally protracted nipples, though, ironically, pregnancy and breastfeeding can also be one of its causes. More to the point of this book, inverted nipple can also be a sign of breast cancer; when this condition is not congenital—meaning that it develops in a woman who has previously had protracted nipples—and it cannot be linked to pregnancy, breastfeeding or injury to the breast, a woman should see a physician for evaluation.

There are also several other benign breast conditions that, while they are physically painless, patients often want to address for emotional and/or aesthetic reasons.

Tubular Breasts

Tubular breasts are a congenital deformity that can affect both women and men and results in breasts that are not fully formed or unequally developed, that are unusually widely spaced, that contain a minimal amount of breast tissue and/or where the areola is enlarged. For women, the condition can cause difficulty with breastfeeding, or even the inability to breastfeed. The cause or causes of this condition are not yet clear, but the condition itself can be successfully and aesthetically addressed through surgery. The caution here is that the procedure is normally more complicated than routine breast augmentation, so the patient should seek out a board certified plastic surgeon who has had specialist training in techniques for tubular breast correction.

Polymastia

Also known as accessory breasts and supernumerary nipples, polymastia is a fairly common condition in which an extra nipple or nipples occur, usually below the line of the normal nipple. These extra nipples are usually small and not well formed, often so much so that they appear to be simply moles, though they can in some cases lactate in breastfeeding women. They can be surgically removed, but in most cases no treatment is needed as they are unrelated to other conditions and do not, when detected in an infant or a child, develop at puberty into breasts.

Poland's Syndrome

Named for Sir Alfred Poland, a nineteenth-century British surgeon, Poland's Syndrome is not specifically a breast condition, but a pattern of malformations that are present at birth, affecting only one side of the body, typically the right. It involves the chest muscle of one side of the body—the muscle that normally attaches to the breastbone is missing—and webbing occurs in the fingers of the same hand. The cause of this condition is not completely understood, but scientists speculate that it may result from the disruption of blood flow around the forty-sixth day of pregnancy, as this is the stage when fetal fingers and chest muscles are developing. Reconstructive surgery is the normal course of treatment—fingers can be separated at an early age; however, breast or chest implants must wait until the patient is a fully-grown adult.

So, as we have seen in this chapter, there are dozens of different sorts of screening techniques and exams, and there are a lot of things that are *not* cancer that can happen with breasts. The medical world continues to work on which sort of screening technique is the best, most effective, least invasive, least toxic way to image a woman's *girls*, but here's a great truth: your own two hands are cheap examination tools and it's really easy to schedule an appointment with yourself to examine your breasts. Just do it!

4

Functional Medicine Approach

Antioxidants

Scrub brushes. That's one way to think about antioxidants—they are mops and polishing cloths and cleaning rags, scrubbing away the dirty, harmful things that can, with stress and age and poor diet and lack of exercise and exposure to ordinary, every day pollutants, accumulate inside of us, just as dust and dirt can pile up on a kitchen floor if its not looked after. Dust and dirt that not only make the floor look unsightly, but the kitchen an unhealthy place in which to prepare food.

Julie

No matter that it was in the month of June when I was diagnosed with breast cancer, at my house we were in the midst of "spring cleaning." But then we are almost always in the midst of some sort of spring cleaning; the task of looking after an intergenerational, two-career family with active teenagers, a big dog, and lots of friends—some of whom, nearly every night of our lives, join us at the dinner table and/or end up after dinner in the family room watching a football game or putting together whatever jigsaw puzzle is spread out on the coffee table—is on-going. Add to this mix the fact that all four members of our nuclear family are on different diets—diets that are, in our case, motivated by health concerns but also informed, as diets almost always are, by personal preferences, some particular brand of I-won't-eat-*that*—and you get the full picture.

Yet it struck me, in those first mornings after my diagnosis, that the effort of keeping a house tidy and ready for company to drop by too often takes priority over keeping our personal houses, our bodies, spick-and-span. Most of us take care of the disorder we can see—the sticky kitchen counter and the dust bunnies under the bed—with relative, if grudging, ease and regularity; but we are frequently not even aware of the disorder we can't see. We deal with the waxy buildup on the coffee table, the rust stains in the bathtub, but where are the TV commercials that might clue us into the really important cleaning chore—the buildup inside of us, the damage caused by the free radicals that we can rightly think of as the biological equivalent of grime and rust.

The concept of ridding—of *cleaning*—the body of free radicals is so integral to both cancer recovery and to cancer prevention, that it is one of the first subjects we talked about in this book, right up front in the Introduction. Let's revisit a little bit of that early discussion before we dive into the specifics of *how* to rid the body of these rabble-rousers. A free radical is a highly toxic, *unstable,* positively-charged atom, molecule or ion. It is unstable because it lacks all of the negatively-charged electrons necessary to complete its structure. Unstable because it wants desperately to complete itself and, like the shady art collector in that wonderful old noir movie, *The Maltese Falcon,* it will wreck every life—every cell—in its path to get what it needs to make its collection of electrons complete.

A free radical steals electrons from other, healthy and whole atoms, molecules and ions in order to stabilize itself. What happens to the victims of the theft, the prey that are left lacking their own complete complement of electrons? Sometimes they will, in turn, become unstable and, in one of those ironic twists of biological fate, end up as free radicals, too. More often they will suffer the damage silently, like a crime victim too scared to fight back, looking to be healed but unable to offer defense as the free radicals run amok inside of us, causing ever more structural damage to our cells, tearing the cells apart atom by atom. Ultimately what will happen is that the free radicals will attack the DNA that is stored within each cell of our body; when the DNA is damaged, that is when cancer begins.

DNA, or deoxyribonucleic acid, is the material found in humans, as well as in most other organisms, that accounts for our hereditary characteristics—why I have my father's nose or you have your Aunt Sophie's smile or your dog has the same color fur as its mother or father. It is present in very nearly every cell of the body, and in two separate places within the cell. If it is located at the center of the cell, or the nucleus, it is known as nuclear DNA; if it is located in the mitochondria—the cell's power plants, where energy is converted into forms that are useable by the cell—it is known as mitochondrial DNA or mtDNA. The genetic code that DNA contains—the code that determines what color hair or what size feet you have, or how tall you are going to be—is stored in the form of chemicals. Here's a detail about those chemicals that's fascinating: there are almost three billion different chemical arrangements currently known that give us our distinctive characteristics, but those arrangements come from only four actual chemicals, or *bases*, in DNA: adenine or (A), guanine or (G), cytosine or (C), and thymine or (T). It is the way these chemicals are arranged in the DNA sequence—GACT or TGAC, for example—that determine our own unique inheritance from our parents', and their parents', and *their* parents' DNA, and so on through all the parents who have come before us in time, chemicals arranging and rearranging themselves within each of our ancestors, over the course of centuries, to assemble themselves today in such a way that results in the unique being that is you.

How can that be? I can imagine you are thinking right now, *Wait just a minute—how can a mere four chemicals arrange themselves in almost three billion different ways?* While genetic science is, of course, not quite this simple, an easier way to think of the arrangement of chemicals along a DNA strand is as if they were the letters of the alphabet—think of how a mere twenty-six letters can be rearranged to make up what is estimated to be the more than quarter million words that make up the English language.

. One of the most important properties of DNA is that it can replicate—and I am not talking here about how your mom's DNA and your dad's joined together and made a human being who, in many ways, replicated *them*. I am talking about the way each strand of DNA that resides in each cell of your body will replicate itself *exactly* in order to create a brand new cell. This is critical because many, though not all, of the cells in our body are constantly dying and replacing themselves, and each new cell must contain the exact same DNA sequence of the cell that it is replacing. While some cells, such as certain nerve and brain cells, are ideally supposed to live and work for us from infancy to old age, others, such as red blood cells, have life spans of about four months. Still others, such as the cells that line the inside or the outside of our bodies—cells that line our stomachs or skin cells, for instance—can live for only twenty hours or so before they are replaced. Think of it: trillions of cells in your body are right now miraculously dividing and replacing themselves precisely, pristinely, identically.

This is not to say that DNA is naturally infallible. Once in about every 100,000,000 instances that a cell prepares to divide and replicate itself, it makes a mistake. In these rare instances, the body is designed to efficiently take care of the error: our bodies contain special DNA repair proteins that detect when a chemical is out of sequence in a DNA strand, and these proteins rush in to swap out the wrong chemical for the right one.

What happens, however, when the DNA is not simply making a rare mistake, but is instead damaged by free radicals? When its telomeres, its big, thick, healthy guards, have been weakened and in their shortened, under-methylated state, are vulnerable to the assault of free radicals? When it is not simply one in 100,000,000 strands of DNA that goof up but DNA that is repeatedly assaulted by a quantity of unstable atoms tearing at the structure of its cell? *What happens is that its capacity to replicate correctly goes awry.* The new cells that are formed have a different arrangement or sequence of the original chemical code—ACTG might become CAGT, as a simple example—and this simple change may have a massive snowballing effect that makes the cell act differently than other cells in which the genetic code is intact. When a cell has replicated frequently enough in this inexact way, the change becomes permanent and is known as a mutation. It is these cells, these damaged or mutated cells, which can cause disease. Cellular damage caused by free radicals is the pathway to rapid aging as well as to a host of illnesses, from autism to Alzheimer's, diabetes and stroke—and cancer.

What caused the cells in my breasts, or your breasts,
to replicate inexactly or mutate, and manifest as our breast cancer? Free radicals.

But what caused the free radicals? Well, for one thing, chemicals.

For many of us, the idea of "chemistry" conjures a caricature of a laboratory with white-coated scientists, mad or otherwise, holding forth over bubbling, steaming vials and vats of strange, Technicolor liquids and gasses. So let's take a moment to ground the idea of chemistry in a friendlier, more everyday context: our own sunny kitchens. If your family is anything like mine, you cook an average of twenty-one meals a week—which means that twenty-one times a week you are in the chemistry lab that is your kitchen, engaging in a chemistry experiment that, depending on your skill level, is more or less successful and pleasing to your family at mealtime. That is, the foods we eat each day are made up of chemicals—the particular chemicals that make broccoli taste and look and smell like broccoli, or eggs like eggs, or that cut of beef like beef. Roasting, sautéing, baking, basting, chilling and marinating, all change the chemical composition of foods. In short, when you cook, what you are doing, at a molecular level, is changing

HOW PESTICIDES AND PETROCHEMICAL FERTILIZERS GET ONTO OUR DINNER PLATES

When I was a little girl, there was a field not far from my house where that beautiful weed, Queen Anne's Lace, grew in abundance. I would often stop by the field after a day of play to pick a bouquet for my mother. One day, my mother asked if I would like to see a trick to turn the naturally creamy-colored heads of the weed into different colors. Well, of course I would! What child wouldn't like a trick like that?

My mother filled several glasses with a little water and, in each one, added a drop or two of food coloring—one glass got blue, one got green, and one got red. Then she divided up the day's bouquet and put a few stems of Queen Anne's Lace into each glass. Soon enough, as the thirsty weeds began to "drink" the water in their "vases"—water infused with the different food colorings—their heads began to turn baby blue, and minty green, and pink.

This little trick—a child's method of turning a handful of weeds into a brightly colored gift for Mom—illustrates vividly what happens to foods that are grown with the use of such substances as pesticides and petrochemical fertilizers: as the plants grow, taking in nutrients from the water and air and soil that surround them, the toxic chemical additives become as much a part of their make-up as the food coloring became a part of those long-ago bouquets I made for my mother.

the cellular structure of foods to make them more palatable, more delicious, more nutritious.

Similarly, our bodies are made up of chemicals that allow us to function—to walk and run, to talk and laugh, to think and learn, to smile when we are happy and give ourselves a scratch when we have an itch. These sorts of chemical compounds are known as *biochemicals*—proteins and enzymes and neurotransmitters and such—but, in spite of their specific, biological names, they act like plain old chemicals in that, when they are confronted by certain outside forces, their cellular structures will change, be damaged or mutate.

It is exposure to the outside forces of other chemicals that does damage to our biochemistry. What sorts of "other chemicals" am I talking about? Chemicals that were used to grow the food we eat and, so, made their way into our bodies by way of a fresh but petrochemically fertilized tomato, or the petrochemically fertilized potato that was used to produce our processed potato chips. Chemicals that make up the sort of standard cleaning products most of us use to mop our kitchen floors or scrub our toilet bowls, uncapped and released into the air for us to breathe in, diluted in water into which we plunge our naked hands and making their way into our bodies by way of the pores in our skin. Chemicals in our makeup and our perfumes, our clothing and our furniture, in the air around us in the form of car exhaust pipes and industrial smokestacks and second-hand smoke. Even *bio*chemicals that our own bodies produce when we are overworked and overwhelmed—that is, under stress.

Another source of those pesky free radicals is electro-magnetic radiation. Though we are only just beginning to recognize them as problems contributing to cancer and other illnesses, UV rays, microwaves, and other sorts of electromagnetic radiation (EMR) can also be a cause of genetic mutation.

Sunlight, the cause of a painful sunburn, is one source of EMR with which we are all familiar. But there are so many other sources that bombard us with radiation these days—the wireless mouse and keyboard of our computer, the router in our home generating Wifi, our cell phones every time we talk or text or use GPS or perform an Internet search, our myriad handheld devices, the microwave oven, the fancy console in our new car that does everything except wipe our tushies for us—these are all sources of electromagnetic energy that gets inside our bodies, assaults our cells and generates free radicals.

How?

There are three acronyms with which we need to be familiar to discuss this next part of the answer: EMR, EMF, and SAR. EMR stands for ElectroMagnetic Radiation that is both emitted and absorbed by charged particles. The phrase 'charged particles' should sound familiar to you—these are atoms that either donate or, like free radicals, are looking for electrons. EMF stands for ElectroMagnetic Field, or an atmosphere created by the charged particles. EMR, the radiation, occupies an EMF, the field. Radiation can be ionizing, such as the radiation that is used to kill cancer cells, meaning that it has enough energy to remove tightly bound electrons from atoms, thus creating ions. It can also be non-ionizing, meaning that it has only enough energy to move atoms around and make them vibrate. Microwaves are one type of non-ionizing EMR, but many if not most of our electronic tools and toys emit microwave EMR to function.

At this point, the next question you will be asking yourself is, *How does EMF relate to me?* Well, the human body absorbs EMR and, as you might expect, just thinking intuitively, absorbing radiation that moves around the atoms inside our bodies might not be a good thing for the human body to be asked to do very often. Since our most significant source of EMR exposure is probably cell phones, I'm going to focus on them as my primary example for the purposes of learning about EMR.

SAR—our final acronym—stands for Specific Absorption Rate. It is very specifically a measure, in watts per kilogram (W/kg), of the EMR absorbed by living tissue when it is exposed to an EMF. In most studies that measure SAR, researchers are looking at brain tissue that has been exposed to the EMR coming off a cell phone in use.

Europe, Australia, and the US, among other countries, have set limits for the amount of SAR that can be emitted from cell phones; interestingly, the European standards are less stringent than the US and Australia but, critically, those standards were created based upon the subject, or recipient, of SAR as a relatively large and weighty adult male, and the object generating the EMR as a 900 mHz phone. The limit set in the US is that no more than 1.6W/kg averaged over 1 gram of tissue should be absorbed by the adult male head and trunk when using a cell phone[53]—but understanding what this standard means is complicated, because when you use your phone, there is variation in how much EMR is emitted depending on *how* and *where* and *who* is using the phone. Texting, for example, emits a lower amount than speaking. The distance you are from a cell tower when the phone is in use is yet another variable that will impact SAR values. What is even more essential to the calculation of SAR in any particular instance, however, is to understand that the absorption rate will be different for humans with less mass and weight than the standard industry subject. There is a much higher SAR in children, as much as 153% more, than in adults.[54] Similarly, a smaller woman has much higher exposure than the large adult male who is the basis for the industry standard.

There has been much discussion about SAR and whether or not it is damaging, and there are discrepancies in the research that has been done. There have been studies that find there are no significant problems and others that find there are issues with the SAR, and these have all been dutifully—and confusingly—reported in the media. What is compelling is that a group of researchers from all over the world came together in 2009 to co-author a paper that discussed the significant concerns about EMR and its potential to cause cancer,

---

53 http://www.fcc.gov/encyclopedia/
specific-absorption-rate-sar-cellular-telephones.

54 http://informahealthcare.com/doi/abs/10.3109/15368378.2011.622827;
http://www.iaeng.org/publication/WCE2010/WCE2010_pp759-763.pdf;
http://www.ncbi.nlm.nih.gov/pubmed/22005525.

especially brain tumors. The authors very specifically discussed the industry's own findings, their bias, and the flaws in their research.[55] They voiced very specific concerns that SAR significantly contributes to causing cancer, especially brain cancer, and offered theories as to how and why it might happen.

Now, this is a book about breasts and breast cancer, so why mention brain cancer? Because the initial SAR research has been conducted on brain tumors. So does that mean that SAR only impacts the brain? If so, then our ta-tas should all be able to breathe a proverbial sigh of relief! But alas, the brain is not, of course, the only area of the body that is exposed to EMR. Our breasts are also exposed—and, in some cases, more directly than in others. There are increasing reports of multifocal breast cancer in very young women. One story I found compelling was presented at a conference I recently attended: a twenty-one-year-old tri-athlete exercised with her cell phone carefully tucked into the special pocket in her sports bras. She developed four different types of breast cancer right below the area where the phone was carried in the center of her chest—a very unusual location for breast tumors.

Now, there are not a lot of double-blinded, placebo-controlled trials looking at breast cancer incidence and cell phone usage—*yet*. And some medical people think that this means there is no evidence-based medicine to support the possibility that cell phone EMR might be contributing to breast cancer. But we need to remember that, similarly, there are no double-

---

55 http://www.radiationresearch.org/pdfs/reasons_us.pdf.

blinded, placebo-controlled trials supporting the use of a parachute to counter the effect of gravity when jumping out of airplanes. In fact, using parachutes has, in terms of the quality of its evidence, to be given an "F" grade by the medical field. This fact was actually published in the medical literature[56]— look at the footnote; I am not making that up. And, yet, given the choice, we would all likely prefer to have access to a parachute if we were jumping out of an airplane, despite the lack of "good medical evidence" that a parachute might be useful on our way down.

So how do we think it happens? How might EMR contribute to breast cancer development? What we know from brain cancer research is that cell phone use increases oxidative stress, augments stress hormones,[57] and damages DNA.[58] And as we've already discussed, these are all things that contribute to breast cancer when they come about through other sources apart from EMR. The solution to these mechanisms of injury is, as it is with the chemicals we discussed above, antioxidants.

We will get to a full discussion of antioxidants in a few paragraphs; for the moment, I'd like to touch on another aspect of EMR—other consequences to the extensive use of cell phones and all of these electronic tools that have less to do with direct cellular damage and more to do with contributing to the stress of living in the electronic age. There are behaviors

---

56 http://www.ncbi.nlm.nih.gov/pubmed/16602356.

57 http://www.sciencedirect.com/science/article/pii/S0928468009000066.

58 http://www.sciencedirect.com/science/article/pii/S0928468009000145.

we have developed as a result of cell phone use that weren't present in days gone by. When I was a child, my house had a rotary phone that had neither call waiting nor an answering machine attached to it. When it rang, we answered it and, if the requested party wasn't in, we took a message—and got in trouble with Mom or Dad if we didn't do it right. Certainly we didn't begin rapidly redialing or frantically texting someone if we didn't get an immediate and instantly gratifying response. But in our electronic age, you don't touch someone else's phone, never mind answer it. It's a given: that phone is always for you—after all, it's *your* phone. We come unglued when the flight attendant tells us we have to turn off our phones on the airplane, and we check our messages and texts as soon as the wheels of the airplane touch the ground again. These individual-use devices that are on our bodies all day long are running our lives. They add a sense of stress and urgency and persuade us with their endless notifications and ringtones that they come first, before any human interaction. They interrupt conversations, they supplant normal communication between people, and they are addictive. When a phone rings or vibrates or beeps, we all stop what we are doing or thinking or saying to be sure that what's happening electronically isn't more important that what we are currently doing in the here and now.

It's gotten a little out of hand, hasn't it?

Actually, "out of hand" is part of the solution. We need to get our electronics off our bodies, out of our hands, away from our heads, and not ranking first in front of everything else in our lives. We need to be able to unplug, disconnect, and get back to breathing, sleeping and living a less frantic, urgent, overdriven lifestyle.

I have a new policy for myself: airplane mode, wherever and whenever possible. Now, this, as a physician on call 24/7, is a challenge, but I still manage it for at least several hours every week. My other policy is using the speakerphone on my cell, to keep my phone away from my head. The corollary to the speakerphone policy is that I've gone back to more private phone conversations; as I've had to leave rooms or wait to place a call until I was alone so that the entire world didn't hear my entire conversation, I've realized how often I was subjecting the world to my half of a phone conversation—a pretty arrogant and rather boring experience for the folks I was with, I think. I owe a lot of folks an apology! Side effects of these new policies? I've been singing at the top of my lungs in my car again. I've had conversations with the lady in the checkout line at the grocery store. I've been *present*.

If you're like most of us, however—or anything like me and my family, you can't afford to stock your kitchen solely with organic foods, and you clean your own house, and you live in a fast-moving, electronic-dependent world where a certain amount of daily environmental[59] as well as emotional pressure is nearly unavoidable. Exposure to free radicals is

---

59 http://deainfo.nci.nih.gov/advisory/pcp/annualReports/pcp08-09rpt/PCP_Report_08-09_508.pdf.

inevitable. They collect in our bodies the way dust piles up on that out-of-the-way end table behind the sofa, or grease accumulates in the hood over the stove. As our mothers instructed us to clean our stove hoods regularly in order to prevent the danger of a grease fire, I'm telling you, in order to prevent cancer, you need to clean up these dangerous free radicals before they can inflict any harm. To help facilitate recovery from cancer, and reverse the damage free radicals have already caused—because, the good news is that it can, indeed, be reversed—you need to clean up those free radicals. To keep your cancer from recurring, you need to *keep* your body clean of free radicals. The question now is, *How?*

Antioxidants.

Antioxidants are the miracle "cleaning solvents" that neutralize free radicals by liberally donating their own electrons to the free radicals, and thus stabilizing them. There are three primary ways to get antioxidants into your body: diet; dietary supplements; and boosting production of or supplementing the body's supply of its natural master antioxidant, *glutathione*.

Diet

Most of us have heard about the U.S. government's old "5 A Day Program" in which we citizens were admonished to eat a minimum of five servings of fruits and vegetables a day. That program has been replaced by "Fruits and Veggies Matter,"[60] a new program that provides not only valuable information about the nutritional importance of fresh produce, but attempts to calculate more exactly the number of servings one needs to eat each day by way of an interactive chart on its home page. The chart's calculations are based on some fairly basic information: your age, your gender, and the level of physical activity you participate in each day. As an experiment, I plugged in my current age (47), my gender (female!), and my level of physical activity (more than 60 minutes a day) and found that, according to the Centers for Disease Control, the institution that runs the program, I should eat two cups of fruits and three of vegetables each day. In contrast, a 57-year-old woman who exercises for only 30 to 60 minutes a day supposedly needs only one and a half cups of fruit and two and a half cups of vegetables.

This is not a bad start, and given how critical nutrition is to the prevention of disease, it seems completely appropriate to me that the effort to promote good nutrition comes to us by way of the Centers for *Disease Control*. But let's remember what we've already talked about in Chapter One: Health is not merely the absence of disease. Official calculations of minimum daily requirements are often just that: recommendations for what we need to do at a minimum to prevent the manifestation of a disease state, rather than guidelines for what we *should* do to experience genuine, robust good health. Because

---

60 http://www.fruitsandveggiesmatter.gov/.

I don't want to just be not sick, I want to have the stamina to smile through a day filled with patient appointments, board meetings, lectures, and family fun, my morning starts out with a big, delicious glass of juice made from whatever fruits and veggies are in the refrigerator—apples, oranges, kale, spinach, celery, parsley and broccoli are a typical combination with a little mint for scrumptious flavor—a bowl of mixed berries, and my favorite, gotta have 'em, lightly sautéed plantains. Lunch is often a salad or a crunchy veggie-laden sandwich—lettuce, tomatoes, cucumbers and sprouts with a little guacamole and sliced turkey on gluten-free bread. Dinner includes at least two cooked vegetables, a salad, and an occasional fruit dessert (on the days when I don't indulge and have a bit of dark chocolate[61]). Some days I try to keep count of how many servings of fruits and veggies I'm eating, but when I make it past eight I usually lose track.

As you can see, I eat a variety of fruits and vegetables, with the emphasis on vegetables, prepared in a variety of ways, both cooked and raw. This leads us to the next important question about the antioxidants we get from our diet: What kind of a mix of fruits and vegetables do we need to maintain or reclaim optimum health? There are three types of antioxidants we can

---

61 The fact that dark chocolate is a potent antioxidant is, in my estimation, a gift from God. *Dark* chocolate is what you want, not milk, as milk can interfere with the body's absorption of chocolate's antioxidants. And remember what I said about official minimum requirements? In the US, a chocolate need contain only 15% cocoa content to be considered dark; read the label on your chocolate bar carefully since, to be an effective antioxidant and not simply an effective way to go up a pant size, it should have a cocoa content of 65% or higher.

get from the foods we eat—carotenoids, isothiocyanates and flavonoids—and human beings need all of them. Fortunately, it's easy to tell what sort of antioxidants are in our produce as the different chemicals that make up each sort of antioxidant manifest in the pigment of the fruit or vegetable. We don't have to keep complicated chemical charts to know we are eating properly; we can, as a general rule, eat by color—by choosing a bright and varied palette for our plates that includes yellow, orange or red, green, and other bright-colored fresh foods.

Carotenoids come in two categories—oxygen-containing molecules like lutein, known as xanthophylls, and the perhaps better-known oxygenated molecules called carotenes, as in beta-carotene. Again, no need to carry a biochemistry book to the supermarket, just choose by color: yellow squash and pineapples, orange carrots and persimmons and apricots for beta-carotene; green leafy vegetables like spinach and kale for lutein; and tomatoes, watermelons and papayas, which are all dense with lycopene, a chemical that enhances the body's ability to put the antioxidants in carotenoids to good use.

Isothiocyanate is the chemical responsible for the green color as well as the flavor and aroma of cruciferous veggies: dark green lettuces, Swiss chard, parsley, chicory, Brussels sprouts. The specific isothiocyanate embedded in broccoli has been shown in some studies to prevent the development of breast cancer so, naturally and almost needless to say, though the absolute scientific proof has yet to be baked into the pudding, I eat a lot of broccoli in my post-cancer life. Breaking the general color rule are isothiocyanates-rich white veggies

JUICING AND ENZYME THERAPY

There are excellent arguments to be made about the value of enzymes and enzyme therapy in treating cancer. Indeed, some chemotherapy drugs, such as asparaginase, are enzyme-based. Enzymes are naturally-occurring proteins that stimulate, and even improve upon or accelerate, the body's biological functions. Digestive enzymes, for example, break foods down so their nutrients can be absorbed more effectively, and metabolic enzymes help to build new cells and repair damaged ones.

Fresh juice is alive with enzymes—but only for about twenty minutes after the juice is extracted from the fruit or vegetable, so juicing at home, minutes before you consume the goodness, is so important. A good juicer has become a standard small appliance in my kitchen; I use a Green Star Twin Gear model—this is a sturdy and reliable, if slightly pricey machine. I like it because it uses flat surfaces to *triturate*, or press, the foods and in that way extract the juice, rather than using blades, so there is a lot less waste.

I cannot emphasize enough the importance of using organic fruits and vegetables for juicing—who wants petrochemical residues mixed in with such a life-giving cocktail? Additionally, I am a huge proponent of juicing *green stuff*—kale, spinach, Swiss chard; veggies that are loaded with iron! I got my hemoglobin level from 7.2 to 10 just two weeks after my surgery *not* by taking iron supplements but by juicing lots of luscious green stuff and drinking one big, sixteen-ounce glass of it every morning; my oncologist nearly dropped his teeth.

like cabbage and cauliflower, and a favorite flavor-enhancer, horseradish.

Flavinoids—which are found in bright-colored foods like raspberries and red cabbage and purple grapes, tree fruits like bananas, grapefruits, lemons and limes, fresh herbs like thyme and dill, as well as teas, chocolate, and red wine—are among the most important foods we humans can eat. They have anti-oxidant and anti-cancer as well as anti-allergy, anti-inflammatory, and antiviral properties. Here's a tip for a delicious way to get at least your minimum requirement of flavonoids: flash frozen fruits and vegetables often have greater nutritional qualities than those that have been picked before their time and left to ripen on the long truck trip to your grocer's produce section; buy a bag of organic, flash frozen raspberries or blueberries to keep in your freezer and scoop half a cup of them right out of the freezer into a bowl of vanilla-flavored coconut milk yogurt—it's like eating dessert for breakfast.

The human body also needs just a small but critical amount of the mineral selenium,[62] which in addition to containing important antioxidant enzymes, also plays a role in boosting the efficiency of the immune system and helps to regulate thyroid function. Selenium, fortunately, is found in many yummy foods—eggs and oatmeal and brazil nuts, some seafood such as tuna (although I choose to avoid the large fish which are often heavily laden with mercury) and codfish, and other proteins such as chicken and beef.

---

62 55 micrograms per day for adults; http://ods.od.nih.gov/factsheets/selenium/.

How these foods are cooked (boiling, for example, decreases the amount of antioxidants in vegetables, so you want to sauté, steam or roast them instead), how often they are eaten (Brazil nuts contain a high amount of selenium and, so, should be enjoyed only occasionally), and how they are combined (serving tomatoes along with avocados or broccoli can increase the absorption of the antioxidants in both) are also keys to antioxidant efficiency. Look in the Resources section at the back of this book for cookbooks and other guides to preparing wholesome anti-cancer meals. I particularly recommend *The Cancer Fighting Cookbook*; it is packed with information on the healing qualities of foods and herbs, but one of the reasons I really love it is its focus on how to prepare flavor-filled meals at a time when chemotherapy and/or radiation may be compromising your taste buds, making many good foods taste bad or seem unappealing.

Dietary Supplements

Eating—putting fruits and vegetables and other foods that contain antioxidants in your mouth, chewing and swallowing and licking your lips—is the way that the body was designed to intake its nutrients, including antioxidants. Therefore, it is just intuitive to understand that the antioxidants we take in by eating are the easiest for our body to put to use. Sadly, the way the bulk of our food is grown today has in many cases significantly *decreased* its nutritional value. Soil depleted of its minerals, which happens when the same crop is grown in the same plot of land year after year, as well as the use of petrochemical fertilizers—two standard practices of big agribusiness—has resulted in vegetables that have, as examples, up to one-fifth less calcium than those same vegetables contained in the 1950s, or a decline in copper content of almost 80%.[63] Produce that has been grown organically, on the other hand, often has a higher nutrient content; relative to the antioxidants we've been talking about, at least one study indicates that organically grown fruits and vegetables contain nearly 40% more antioxidants than those that have been grown at factory farms.[64]

Organic produce, however, is generally more expensive, and therefore not always within a family's budget, and it is not readily available in all areas of the country. I recommend that folks try hard to eat at least the dirty dozen foods as organically as possible. Beyond that, to get what our stressed bodies need when we're dealing with cancer: vitamin supplements to the rescue!

The four most important vitamin supplements to incorporate in your antioxidant, anti-cancer diet are vitamin A, vitamin C, vitamin E, and, critically, vitamin D.

---

63 http://depthome.brooklyn.cuny.edu/anthro/faculty/mitrovic/davis_2009_food_nutrient.pdf.

64 http://www.drweil.com/drw/u/WBL02077/Organic-Foods-Have-More-Antioxidants-Minerals.html.

THE DIRTY DOZEN

All vegetables are not created equal. Some are more nutri-tious than others and, I dare say, however big a fan I am in general, some are more delicious, too. Alas, in our modern, big-agriculture world, some are *much* less equal. Because of such things as vulnerability to insect and fungus infestation, some crops are more heavily sprayed with pesticides and those are the ones we want to avoid. This is a list of the top twelve most important sources of antioxidants to buy organic.

1. **Apples.** Because so many different insects and kinds of fungus threaten apple harvests, this is one of the most heavily sprayed crops in the world. More than forty different pesticides are used to combat these threats and, not coincidentally, traces of these pesticides can also be found in applesauce, apple juice, and other apple products. If organic apples aren't available to you—and even considering that apple rinds contain a lot of nutrients—we recommend that you peel them before eating.

2. **Bell peppers.** In every sweet, antioxidant color they come in, they can come laced with over fifty different pesticides. There is no substitute, so go organic with this fruit.

Vitamin A, in addition to being a fine antioxidant, impacts your vision, bone growth, and immune function. But we rarely take vitamin A tablets because it has been traditionally thought to be quite toxic in excess. It is interesting to note, at the time of writing this book, the medical world's approach to vitamin A is getting a new look with fresh eyes, but it is not time to change our recommendations on doses and forms of vitamin A—*yet*. Instead, we currently supplement vitamin A by taking *beta-carotene*, which is a precursor to vitamin A—that is, the body converts beta-carotene into the vitamin A it needs. Dietary sources include liver, whole milk (for those who can tolerate casein in their diets), egg yolks, spinach, carrots, cantaloupes, cabbages, kiwis, kale and certain enriched cereals. Beta-carotene is important not only for cancer patients, but especially for young children and, as alcohol depletes the body of vitamin A, alcoholics.

Vitamin C is also not just an antioxidant—it promotes healing, and extra doses are recommended for folks who are recovering from surgery or injury; it is important to the health of your skin, bones, and connective tissue; and it helps the body to absorb iron. Extra vitamin C is often recommended for smokers, burn victims, and women who are pregnant or breastfeeding.

Vitamin E multitasks as well, functioning as an antioxidant as well as playing a role in regulating the body's metabolic processes and immune function.

Vitamin D is a subject about which I could absolutely rhapsodize! It is still sort of astonishing to me that the ben-

3. **Celery.** USDA tests have detected over sixty different pesticides on celery samples. If you can't find organic celery, try radishes in the crudité tray.

4. **Potatoes.** The lowly potato—and the French fries and chips and Thanksgiving side dish of mashed that are made from it: over thirty-five different pesticides are used on this crop. For fresh, try substituting sweet potatoes and yams if you can't find organic. As for processed foods—those sometimes irresistible fast food fries included—this pesticide contamination is one more reason you're better off resisting.

5. **Spinach.** Fifty different pesticides have been detected in both fresh and frozen spinach, and the canned variety doesn't fare much better. Popeye would weep. This is a must-buy-organic vegetable.

6. **Lettuce.** Right up there with spinach and its fifty different pesticides. If you can't find organic, it is better to forego the salad and go with greens like broccoli, green beans or asparagus.

7. **Kale.** For a leafy green—and a particularly hardy one to boot—it is almost as contaminated as spinach and lettuce. Try Swiss chard instead if you can't find organic.

8. **Strawberries.** Strawberries are susceptible to fun-

efits of this vitamin—and the perils associated with the lack of it—are not more widely known and acted upon. Vitamin D is necessary to the body's absorption of calcium, which is, in turn, essential for good bone health. It is also needed for the efficient functioning of the immune, nervous, and muscle systems. And, research suggests, having adequate stores of it in the body is part of what can help to prevent breast cancer.[65]

But how much of each of these vitamins do *you* need? How much do you need to maintain vibrant health, and how much do you need as a cancer patient and, then, as a cancer survivor? Regrettably, there is no one easy answer. The current RDA (recommended daily allowance) for vitamin E is 15 IU for adult men and 12 for adult women. For vitamin C the RDA is 60 mg per day, and for vitamin D it is a paltry 22.5 IU for an adult woman who is not breastfeeding. These are, in reality, far too low for most adults and, because beta-carotene is converted into vitamin A in the body, there is no current set requirement at all for this particular vitamin! So, how do you know how much to take? Well, how tall are you and how much do you weigh? What does your normal diet consist of? How much exercise do you get? What other supplements or medications are you taking—because, for example, if you take blood thinners regularly, your doctor may recommend lower doses of vitamin E, or even avoiding it altogether.

---

65 http://health.ucsd.edu/news/releases/Pages/2013-01-24-breast-cancer-linked-to-vitamin-d-levels.aspx.

gus and, in turn, farmers spray this crop heavily to keep their crop "healthy." Substitute pineapples, bananas, and kiwis if you can't buy organic.

9. **Blueberries.** And cranberries and cherries. While the latter two often contain less than the fifty different pesticides that are used on blueberries, they are often just as contaminated.

10. **Peaches.** Fresh, juicy, delicious peaches! It's almost a crime that over sixty pesticides have been found on this gorgeous fruit! But if you can't find organic, we recommend you substitute a different fruit, or try using canned peaches as they tend to contain less pesticides than the fresh, non-organic fruit.

11. **Nectarines.** Imported nectarines are one of the most highly contaminated fruits you'll find in your grocer's produce section. Domestically grown ones fare much better, but still we'd recommend substituting if you can't find organic. Pineapples and mangos are a better choice.

12. **Grapes.** Over thirty different pesticides have been detected on grapes of all varieties. Ditto the raisins that are made from grapes. And, you won't be stunned to find out, in the wine that is also made from them. They are so contaminated as a crop that we recommend only organic grapes and grape products.

1 To stay abreast of each year's new Dirty Dozen list, go here: http://www.thedailygreen.com/healthy-eating/eat-safe/dirty-dozen-foods#fbIndex1.

Actual doses of each of these are difficult to recommend without individual consultation. In general, most physicians will not worry if their patient takes 1000 mg of vitamin C, 200 IU of vitamin E, 2500 IU of vitamin A, and 1000 IU of vitamin D on a daily basis. It is quite possible to get much more than these base levels by drinking a big glass of good organic juice in the morning, so if you are supplementing, it's important to consider signs of too high doses of these vitamins. Vitamin C in very, very high doses will cause diarrhea. Too much vitamin A will cause a fine red rash from head to foot. And there will be bruising and prolonged bleeding with high doses of vitamin E. Interestingly, too much vitamin D3 is a situation we really haven't confidently described in the medical literature. This could be because we were really designed to be outside, naked, 24/7.

I used liberal doses of vitamins and supplements whenever I wasn't feeling nauseated during my chemo, a treatment I underwent *before* my surgery, and I vividly remember negotiating with Ankit about stopping some of them, specifically the omegas and the vitamin E before I went into the operating room. He asked for two weeks off them before surgery, but I wanted no more than three days. We settled at a week off to decrease the likelihood of bleeding too much and too long. I suspect that, though he never yelled at me because he is quite possibly the very nicest surgeon to walk the earth, I may have made his work harder on the day of my surgery by being so stubborn.

Glutathione

Did you ever hear this old joke? Guy walks into a doctor's office, sits down in the chair in front of the doctor's desk, lifts up one leg, grabs his foot and wraps his ankle around the back of his head. "Doc," he says when he's all tangled up, "it hurts when I do this." "Well," the doctor replies, "don't do that."

Sound medical advice, as far as I can tell, loaded with common sense, and effective. Generally the things we do that cause us pain are things we are not supposed to be doing, or that we aren't prepared to do. If the guy in our joke was a yoga master then, sure, one might expect him to be able to twist into that heel-behind-head position, but you and I—and even though yoga is one of my preferred forms of exercise—probably can't pull off a move like that. Pain is one of the body's primary ways of communicating with itself: the nerves say, Hey, there's a terrific pain down here in my foot, and the brain responds, almost instantaneously, by contracting muscles that move the foot away from the bedpost it has stubbed up against or the bee it has stepped on. Sometimes it takes the brain a little longer to figure out what's causing the discomfort. A friend recently called for some medical advice: her mouth was itchy and tingling, her lips were swollen, her tongue was raw and her gums were inflamed—she couldn't even smile without great distress. What was wrong, she urgently wanted to know. Off hand, I couldn't tell her, so I asked her some questions starting with might she have eaten something lately that wasn't part of her normal diet? Could she be having an allergic reaction to some new food? No, she assured me, she hadn't gone on any culinary adventures lately; that couldn't be it. Besides, she said, it had been going on for three days and it was getting worse by the day, she couldn't even brush her teeth without a terrible burning sensation… That was where she stopped. Cold. She had switched toothpastes three days before, from her normal mint-flavored variety to one that was flavored with the oils of cinnamon and clove. Two days after quitting the new toothpaste, she was once again able to smile.

Our bodies also tell us *to do* certain things. They tell us to eat when we're hungry and sleep when we're tired. The cravings that pregnant women are (sometimes unjustly) famous for may be the body's way of communicating that it needs the nutrients found in those sometimes peculiar foods—Natalie Portman, a dedicated vegan, reported that during her pregnancy she started to eat cheese and eggs because her body told her it needed them. Nail biters—Princess Di was a famous one—might not just have a nervous habit; their bodies might be yearning for calcium, and that's what fingernails, and toenails, are made of.

What happens, though, when your body needs something and you don't know it? When the fact that a certain material exists in the body is such a new one, and so relatively unstudied that its impact on human health has not yet been wholly acknowledged by the established medical community? Those of us in the autism community have understood for many years the role that glutathione plays in recovering these kids from their disorder but, though it was first discovered in 1888 and there are now nearly 90,000 references to it in the U.S. National Library of Medicine of the National Institutes for Health, many traditional medical practitioners remain either unaware of its benefits in the treatment of cancer, or hesitant to recommend its use because it has not yet become standard practice.

Again, however, I stress the disconnect between what has or has not yet been proved through strenuous research and what actually works in practical, clinical practice. Here is what you need to know about glutathione as it relates to cancer patients:

- **glutathione** is the body's homemade master antioxidant—it is as essential to the sustenance of life as air and water;

- **cancer is caused** when DNA is damaged by free radicals;

- **free radicals** run amok when the body does not have enough antioxidants to protect the DNA in its cells;

- **cancer patients** almost invariably[66] present with reduced glutathione levels and extraordinary oxidative stress.[67]

---

66 It is important to note that lung cancer may be one of the few cancers for which glutathione treatment is not recommended. http://www.ncbi.nlm.nih.gov/pubmed/8687095.

67 http://www.ncbi.nlm.nih.gov/pubmed/21811816.

Glutathione, in biochemical lingo, is a tripeptide, meaning that it has three components—cysteine, glutamic acid and glycine—and it comes in two forms, an Oxidized form, GSSG—which I choose to remember alliteratively as "Out-of-commission," and a Reduced, or, again alliteratively, "Ready-to-go" form, GSH. The GSH foils free radicals (as well as other ROS—reactive oxygen species, like peroxides) by donating its electrons to make them stable. In the process of losing its electrons in this way, it is converted to GSSG. The percentage of GSH in a healthy body is about 90 to the GSSG's 10 and, indeed, the ratio of glutathione in its reduced form and its oxidized form is sometimes used to measure a patient's level of cellular toxicity or oxidative stress. Glutathione's purpose in the body is much easier to explain—it protects the cell's DNA and, thus, prevents disease—and there is no other substance in the world that does this job better. The logical appeal is, again, plain:

● **Glutathione** protects DNA.

● **Damaged DNA** causes cancer.

● **Cancer patients** typically have low glutathione levels.

And the conclusion is just as clear:

● **Supplement** cancer patients' glutathione.

Glutathione can be given to a patient in several ways. Tablets, which are to be taken by mouth, for example, though studies have shown that glutathione is not easily absorbed orally by the body, even when taken sublingually (holding the pill under the tongue until it is slowly dissolved) as is often recommended. There are also glutathione patches, which are worn on the skin, but do not work the way most patches do—that is, transdermally, with a substance being absorbed through the skin; glutathione patches are placed on acupuncture points on the body and work by reflecting infrared light frequencies in the body. I won't discount the science out of hand—these patches are homeopathic remedies and I have seen certain homeopathic treatments work very well— but even their manufacturers state that the patches are useful for cancer *prevention*; *curing* cancer is a whole different ball game.

I have found glutathione injections and infusions to be the most effective method of dispensing the supplement. When a supplement is taken orally, it has to be processed by the digestive system before it can get into the body to do its good work. Gastric juices can dilute the efficacy of the supplements, and for those whose digestive systems are compromised, such as my autism patients, 80% of whom suffer from digestive problems, supplements that are given orally can be rendered completely useless. Injections and infusions deliver the glutathione directly into the blood stream where it can begin its work unmolested and immediately.

The infusions are relatively painless and quick—one quick prick of a needle that even my young autism patients come not to mind in relation to how good they feel after an infusion. Depending on the dose, they can take as little as five minutes, or up to half an hour, and even my busy NFL players make the time to be infused regularly.

In my practice, each infusion for each patient is custom-made. I mix up a special "cocktail" that includes glutathione and can also include vitamins such as B and/or C, and minerals such as magnesium, depending on what the patient needs *that day*. Remember, what the body needs on any given day, in any given circumstance, is dynamic, and functional medicine takes that into account. Is one of my young patients coming down with a cold? She might get a little extra vitamin C to fight the infection. Is one of my football players feeling especially fatigued? A little more vitamin B for energy.

I had been prescribing glutathione infusions for my patients for many years, and though the nurses in my office would see me winding down over the course of a long week and offer to give me an infusion myself, I rarely took them up on the offer in my pre-cancer life. I had too much to do to sit still for half an hour, right? While I was fighting cancer, and now, in my post-cancer life, glutathione infusions are just part of the weekly routine.

Where can you get a glutathione infusion? Unlike tablets and patches, injections and infusions require a prescription. Increasingly, integrative and functional medicine physicians are experienced in using glutathione infusions. See the Resource section at the back of this book for suggestions on how to locate an integrative or functional medical specialist.

One more thing: I have been fascinated by the oncology offices that have adamantly warned patients to avoid antioxidants during chemotherapy. This does seem to be declining, quite possibly because the next generation of chemotherapeutic agents that is being developed is reported to be antioxidants!

5

Assessing and Managing Breast Health Risks

Lots of my patients have told me that, upon
diagnosis, one of the first thoughts that
went through her mind was, Why?

Let me be clear: the question is, Why?
It is rarely ever, Why me?

Ankit

Warren Buffett is an American business magnate and philanthropist, the first or second or third richest person in the world—depending on who's adding up the bank account and in which year—and he is regarded globally as one of the most successful investors of all time. As an investor, he is a person who knows a thing or two about risk. "Risk is a part of God's game, alike for men and nations," Mr. Buffett has said, and he's right in the most fundamental sense possible. Simply living, simply taking part in everyday life, involves chance at every turn—perhaps more chance than we're comfortable admitting, but we still make efforts to mitigate it. We may have never slipped in the tub, but we still use a bathmat. We may live in a safe neighborhood, but we still lock our doors at night. We may not have had a fender bender in a decade, but we still carry car insurance. For most of us, taking these sorts of precautions is second nature—even part of a cultural wisdom that comes from collectively having already assessed the risks involved in such activities as bathing and driving and passed on what we can do to lessen them.

More basically, we lock our doors at night and carry car insurance because we *know* to do them. Knowing how to prevent disease, however, is still rather new as cultural wisdom goes. To be sure, we've got some of the big culprits cornered—pretty much everyone knows that smoking cigarettes or eating trans-fats is like taking a highway that leads directly to the hospital—but what about other disease risks? What are some of the more nuanced actions we can take to prevent illness? And, in an Internet world cluttered with sometimes questionable advice, how can we tell correct information from the merely sensational or the downright wrong?

As Mr. Buffett has also said, "Risk comes from not knowing what you're doing." Though he was probably talking about things like analyzing a company's capital structure—its debt/ equity ratio, for example—before one invests in it, he could just as easily have been a doctor talking to a patient about staying healthy: your chances of preventing disease are in many ways proportional to how much you know about disease prevention. In this chapter, I'm going to rather comprehensively cover the known risk factors for breast cancer, debunking a few of them along the way, so you'll have a better understanding of how to preserve—and restore—breast health.

Breast Cancer Risk Factors and Predictors

A "risk factor" is simply something that has the potential to predict something else. Let's go back to our example of driving a car. Every day when you drive to work, for instance, there is a risk that you will come home with a dent in your fender, but there are steps that you can take—and that your insurance company would highly commend—to minimize the risk: making sure your car is in good working order, the treads on your tires aren't worn, you aren't chatting on the cell phone and you are wearing your seatbelt, for example. Just because you're wearing your seatbelt, however, doesn't mean that another driver won't rear end you on the off ramp; but it does mean that you're more likely to walk away from the accident without serious injury. The same is true for disease: just because you have a risk factor does not mean you will get the disease and, conversely, just because you don't have a risk factor doesn't mean you won't.

In terms of disease, there are two kinds of risk factors: those you can't change and those you can. Alzheimer's generally afflicts older people, and none of us can change the fact that aging is part of life. Your risk of Alzheimer's increases just because you get older, and that isn't something we can change. Smoking cigarettes, on the other hand, is a known risk factor for lung cancer and smoking is a behavior a person *can* change. Knowing what your risks are can help you change the behaviors that may have contributed to your illness—and changing those risky behaviors can not only help to keep you well once you have regained your health, but changing them immediately, as soon as you are diagnosed, can be an effective part of the treatment phase of your recovery. It goes without saying that never engaging in risky behaviors in the first place is the ultimate in disease prevention, but very few of us have lived in hermetically sealed environments since the time before we were even born. The trick to easing risk then becomes being able to forgive ourselves for having had bad habits in the past— instead of focusing on the damage that may have been done to our bodies by years of consuming McDonald's French fries, let's celebrate that we have overcome our craving for them!

Risk Factors We Cannot Change

- **Age.** The chance of getting breast cancer increases with age. According to the National Cancer Institute, a woman under the age of thirty-nine has a 1 in 233 chance of being diagnosed with breast cancer. But in the next decade of her life, that risk increases to 1 in 69. Over the next decade, that risk increases once again, to 1 in 42, and women over the age of sixty-nine have a risk factor of 1 in 29.[68] These numbers should, by the way, be making you shake your head and blink and re-read. They are, in fact, appallingly high.

- **Gender.** The chances of a woman getting breast cancer is 100 times greater than that of a man. This is not because, in the vast majority of cases, women simply have more

---

68 http://www.cancer.gov/cancertopics/factsheet/detection/ probability-breast-cancer.

breast tissue than men, and hence a greater number
of cells with the potential to contract the disease, but
because they have more of the female hormones estrogen and progesterone—both of which promote growth,
including the growth of tumors—to which their breast
tissue is constantly exposed over the course of a lifetime.

● **Family history.** According to the Centers for Disease
Control, a woman who has just one immediate, or *first-
degree* female relative—a mom, a sister, or a daughter—
who has had breast cancer has a "moderate" increase in
risk for breast cancer herself. A woman who has two or
more such close relatives who have experienced breast
cancer, however, has a "strong" possibility of developing
the disease herself. Further, the risk is increased by other
factors: if those relatives received their diagnoses before
the age of fifty, or if the diagnoses involved both breasts,
or if the relative who received the diagnosis was male.[69]

● **Personal history.** A *recurrence* of cancer is defined as
cancer that has been successfully treated but is detected
again after a cancer-free period of time. A recurrence
can be *local*, meaning that it occurs near the site of the
previous tumor, or in tissue or skin near the site of the
previous tumor if the breast has been removed; *regional*,

---

69 http://www.cdc.gov/genomics/resources/diseases/breast_ovarian_cancer/
risk_categories.htm.

meaning, in the case of breast cancer, that it occurs, for
example, in the lymph nodes near the initially affected
breast; and *distant*, meaning, in the case of breast cancer, that it recurs in the other breast. The American
Cancer Society attaches a 3- to 4-fold increase in risk
for the development of new cancer in women who have
already had a breast cancer experience.[70] The good news
is that real progress is being made in this area. Above and
beyond the growing understanding that adopting healthy
lifestyle choices can significantly reduce the chance of
recurrence, new drugs that can be used to help prevent
recurrence are being developed and tested all the time,[71]
and new therapies, such as psychological intervention,
that have proved effective in reducing recurrence are
being studied and introduced.[72]

● **Dense breast tissue.** Women whose breast composition contains more glandular than fatty tissue are said to
have "dense breast tissue." This is not, of itself, a condition that should cause alarm, but the more fibrous tissue
does make traditional mammograms more difficult to
interpret. Some studies are showing that, for women who

---

70 http://www.cancer.org/cancer/breastcancer/detailedguide/
breast-cancer-risk-factors.

71 For example, a 2010 study shows that anastrozole is better than the more commonly prescribed tamoxifen at preventing recurrence; http://www.cancer.gov/
clinicaltrials/results/summary/2004/ataci204.

72 http://www.medscape.org/viewarticle/583889.

have dense breasts, digital mammography may be a more
effective regular screening option.[73]

- **Race and ethnicity.** White women have the highest
  incidence of breast cancer, black women the second highest, Hispanic women the third, followed by Asian/Pacific
  Islander women at fourth, and then, with the lowest risk,
  American Indian and Alaska Native women.[74] Within
  these general statistics, however, are nuances: white
  women, for example, are more likely to be diagnosed
  with small, local tumors, while black women are more
  likely to be diagnosed with larger or distant tumors.[75]
  Why is this? It may be due to breast biology, or specific
  environmental risk factors, but likely it is not the rate at
  which breast cancer early-screening tools are used by different ethnic groups—the most current statistics available
  show that by a reed-thin margin, a higher percentage of
  black women than white have annual mammograms.[76]

- **Genetic risk factors.** *Hereditary breast cancer* is caused
  by a mutant gene that is passed from parent to child.
  Approximately 5% to 10%—though by some estimates
  as much as 27%—of all breast cancer incidence is

---

73 http://www.mayoclinic.com/health/mammogram/AN01137.

74 http://www.cdc.gov/features/dsbreastcancertrends/.

75 http://www.ncbi.nlm.nih.gov/pubmed/15224974.

76 http://www.cdc.gov/cancer/breast/statistics/screening.htm.

MALE BREAST CANCER

Breast cancer is an equal opportunity disease—not only women, but men can get it, too, although in much smaller numbers. Women get breast cancer at about 100 times the rate that men do: the American Cancer Society estimates that in 2013, about 2,500 new cases of male breast cancer will be diagnosed, and that a little over 400 men will die from the disease.

Other than the rarity of this cancer in men, what men and what women experience when diagnosed with breast cancer is quite similar. As with the disease in women, most men who are diagnosed with breast cancer are older, the diagnostic and treatment tools are the same, men who inherit BRCA mutations from a parent are at greater risk, and early diagnosis dramatically improves the prognosis. Here's the rub: because the awareness of men's breast cancer in no way approaches that of women's, many men don't even realize that they *could* get the disease. Consequently, men will dismiss or ignore the warning signs of breast cancer; while men have little breast tissue in comparison to women, and it is easier for them and/or their doctors to detect a breast lump, because the possibility of cancer is so off their radar, by the time they see a medical professional about a lump the cancer has often already spread to surrounding tissues or lymph nodes.

Unfortunately, another reason men will sometimes delay seeing a doctor about a suspicious breast lump is self-consciousness about changes in their breast area and/or because they feel embarrassed about presenting with a 'feminine' disease. It is worth repeating at his juncture: early diagnosis means a better prognosis.

Symptoms of male breast cancer are:

1. A change in the size or shape of the breast

2. A lump or thickening in the breast, often painless

3. Dimpling or puckering, redness or scaling in the skin covering the breast, and redness or scaling around the nipple area

4. A nipple that begins to invert, or turn inward

5. Discharge from the nipple

The good news is that it is very common to find out the breast lump is not cancer but *gynecomastia*, a benign breast condition that manifests as an enlargement of the breast resulting from a hormone imbalance. A hormone imbalance can be brought on by events such as puberty, conditions such as obesity, or a wide variety of both prescription medication and non-prescription drugs. Usually, unless there is pain involved (as there can be in rare cases), no further treatment is needed.

hereditary.[77] Probably the best-known genetic mutations thought to be responsible for hereditary breast
cancer involve the BRCA1 and BRCA2 genes—or *br*east
*ca*ncer susceptibility gene *1* and *br*east *ca*ncer susceptibility gene *2*—though not all breast cancers are caused by
these genes. BRCA1 and BRCA2 mutations are currently
thought to account for only about half of the cases of
hereditary breast cancer,[78] and "the consensus is building
that there is no single strong breast cancer gene left to be
discovered…it's most likely that there are many different
genes, and that each may account for a small fraction of
the remaining families."[79] BRCA1 and BRCA2 belong to
a class of genes known as tumor suppressors. Some tumor
suppressor genes or, more accurately, tumor suppressor
proteins, work by inhibiting the reproduction of cells that
contain damaged DNA—and, remember, it is the reproduction and/or mutation of damaged DNA that causes
cancer. Other tumor suppressor genes work by causing
apoptosis, or programmed cell death, when cell damage
cannot be repaired by the special repair proteins we spoke
of in Chapter Four. It is when the BRCA1 or BRCA2
cells have mutated, and these mutations are passed from
parent to child, that the incidence of breast cancer, as
well of ovarian, cervical, uterine, pancreatic and a range

---

77 http://www.genome.gov/10000507.

78 http://www.genome.gov/10000532#al-1.

79 Ibid.

of other cancers, may increase. It is possible to be tested for the BRCA 1 and BRCA 2 genes—usually a blood sample is drawn and technicians use various methods, including checking protein levels, to determine a result. Currently no standard exists to definitely determine whether a woman—or a man, who can carry these gene mutations as well—should have these genetic tests. A family history of breast cancer is used as a guideline, as is ethnicity for women of Ashkenazi, or Eastern European, Jewish descent.[80] But *should* you be tested? In the U.S., 1 in 8, or about 12%, of women will develop breast cancer during her lifetime, but nearly 80% of women with a BRCA1 or BRCA2 mutation will develop breast cancer.[81] That statistic is a compelling reason to be tested if you fit family history or ethnic parameters. The caution is to approach the test understanding that, while a *positive* result indicates a higher risk for developing cancer, it does not mean that a woman will absolutely get cancer. I also highly recommend that women who opt for this testing do so with the guidance of an experienced genetic counselor who can help them interpret the test and decide on a course of action.

---

80 Approximately 2.65 percent of the Ashkenazi Jewish population carries a BRCA1 or BRCA2 mutation, as opposed to 0.2% of the general population. http://www.genetichealth.com/BROV_GEN_of_BROV_In_ASHJ.shtml.

81 http://www.breastcancer.org/risk/factors/genetics.jsp.

● **Certain benign breast conditions.** In Chapter Three
we wrote about several benign breast conditions that are
not, or are highly unlikely to be, risk factors for breast
cancer. There are other breast conditions as well, usually
benign, that have the potential to be of greater concern.
Usually these conditions are divided into three categories,
based on how they impact the potential risk for cancer.

  • *Non-proliferative lesions* do not indicate breast cancer
  risk, or do so only in a very small percentage of cases.
  Lesion is a broadly defined term meaning any abnormality in the tissue of any organism, and such an
  abnormality can be caused by any event that damages
  the tissue—trauma, for example, or non-cancerous
  disease. *Proliferative* means that the lesion grows,
  or spreads, at a rapid rate. So, the first category of
  benign breast conditions involve lesions that are *non-*
  proliferative, or do not grow or spread. Fibrocystic
  breasts and breast cysts, two of the common benign
  breast conditions we spoke of in Chapter Three, are
  included in this category.[82]

  • *Proliferative lesions without atypia* slightly (1 to 2
  times) increase the risk of breast cancer. *Atypia* is
  medical jargon for tissue with an increased or excessive presence of abnormal cells that may or may not

---

82 Types of non-proliferative breast lesions: adenosis (non-sclerosing); duct ectasia;
fat necrosis; fibroadenoma (simple); fibrocystic breasts; hamartoma; hemangioma;
hyperplasia (mild); lipoma; mastitis (breast infection); neurofibroma; papilloma
(single); Phyllodes tumor.

become cancerous. This second category then—proliferative but *without* atypia—encompasses lesions
that have demonstrated the ability to grow or spread,
but do not include an excessive presence of suspicious
cells in their make up. This second category, like the
first, can include fibroadenomas, in this case referred
to as *complex* fibroadenomas, which contain abnormal but not cancerous growths or cells.[83]

- *Proliferative lesions with atypia* strongly (4 to 5 times)
increase the risk of breast cancer.[84] This category, as
the name suggests, includes lesions that are prolifer-
ating, or growing, and that do contain an excessive
number of abnormal but not cancerous cells. The
two terms you will hear associated with this category
are "atypical ductal hyperplasia" or ADH, meaning a
growth containing an excessive amount of abnormal
cells that is located in the breast duct or ducts, and
"atypical lobular hyperplasia" or ALH, meaning a
growth containing an excessive amount of abnormal
cells is located in the lobe or lobes of the breast. For
women who have a family history of breast cancer, a
diagnosis of ADH or ALH is of particular concern as
the risk of breast cancer increases. Even in these cases,

---

83 Types of proliferative breast lesions without atypia: adenosis (sclerosing); ductal
hyperplasia (without atypia); fibroadenoma (complex); papillomas (multiple;
referred to as papillomatosis); radial scar.

84 *http://www.breastsurgeons.org/statements/PDF_Statements/Ductal_Cell.
pdf.*

however, the diagnosis is not a clear indication that breast cancer will result. In fact, a 2008 study conducted at the Mayo Clinic found that, as a predictor of breast cancer, the Gail model, a statistical model that is commonly used by clinicians to calculate the possibility that a woman will develop breast cancer, is not accurate when used to evaluate women with atypical hyperplasia.[85] What such a diagnosis does mean is that the woman should discuss with her doctor the plan they are going to follow for careful, more frequent screenings in the future.

● **Lobular carcinoma in situ (LCIS).** *In situ* is a Latin term that translates, literally, as "in position." In this case, it means abnormal cells in position, or situated, in the lobules, or milk glands, of the breast. And, while *carcinoma* is, indeed, the medical term used to describe cancerous growths, LCIS is not cancer. It is, however, an indication that a woman may be at increased risk of breast cancer, and that she and her doctor should discuss increased breast cancer screening and other preventative measures.

● **Onset and cessation of menstrual periods.** The hormones estrogen and progesterone, as we have said before, promote growth. Women who begin menstruating

85 http://www.mayoclinic.org/news2008-rst/5059.html.

early—before the age of twelve—or cease menstruating late—after the age of fifty-five—have a greater lifetime exposure to these growth-promoting hormones and it is thought that this is why women at either extreme of the spectrum for menstrual onset develop breast cancer more frequently.

● **Chest radiation.** Radiation therapy saves lives—and it is one of the viable treatment options for breast cancer that we'll discuss in Chapter Eight—but it can also cause other health complications. Women who have had, as children or as young adults, radiation therapy to the chest area to treat a previous cancer, such as Hodgkin disease or non-Hodgkin lymphoma, have a greatly increased risk of developing breast cancer. Let me emphasize the timing of the treatment: the increased risk appears to be most significant when the previous, chest-area radiation therapy was administered when the women were children or were young adults or, in short, *when breast tissue was still developing*. Alternatively, there is some evidence that radiation treatment to the chest area that is administered after a woman is forty or older has no impact on her risk of developing breast cancer. I also want to note here that the risk of cancer seems to be lessened for those women who, concurrently with previous chest-area radiation treatment, also underwent chemotherapy. This is thought to be attributable to the fact that certain chemo drugs will stop the production of growth hormones (estrogen and progesterone) for the period of therapy—the patient's exposure to these hormones is lessened, as is the risk of breast cancer.

- **Diethylstilbestrol (DES) exposure.** Diethylstilbestrol, DES or, formerly, BAN stilboestrol, is a synthetic form of estrogen that was developed in 1938—and its long history is also a controversial one. Notably, to the point of this book, in the 1940s on into the 1970s, it was given, off-label, to pregnant women who had a history of miscarriage, as it was thought to help them carry the pregnancy to full term. In spite of an absence of evidence that it actually served its intended, off-label purpose— evidence that began accumulating in the early 1950s—it wasn't until 1971 that the FDA began advising doctors not to prescribe it for pregnant women. Among its other, more spurious off-label uses was as a prescription to combat "excessive height" in prepubescent girls; from the 1950s through the 1970s, and in spite of what was by then a clear link to cancer—not to mention a later link to the growth of rare vaginal tumors in women who had been exposed to the drug in utero—it was prescribed for young girls who were thought to be growing too tall! In 1997, the last remaining manufacturer of the drug, Eli Lilly, stopped making it, but its impact is on-going: DES daughters and DES sons, as the children who were exposed to this drug while in utero are known, have an increased risk of infertility, genital abnormalities, poten-

PROPHYLACTIC MASTECTOMIES

In the late spring of 2013, the actress and humanitarian Angelina Jolie made a courageous revelation that changed the way many women will deal with their breast cancer—or how they will react when they come into knowledge that they may develop breast cancer. She revealed she had had a double prophylactic mastectomy.

This is a book about the prevention and treatment of breast cancer; I believe the medical and ethical debate behind that most personal decision to undergo a prophylactic mastectomy or mastectomies deserves a book unto itself. Still, it is a crossroads that more and more of us will come to as genetic testing for the BRCA genes becomes more and more commonplace, so I'll relate two personal stories that may offer comfort and insight to women standing at the juncture.

I am BRCA negative but, when I found my cancer, one of the first things I flashed on was my mother, a thirty-year cancer survivor. I thought of all the mammograms mom has continued to have over the years. And the biopsies she has had to have on the two occasions when her mammography results indicated there might be a recurrence of her cancer. I remembered how we held our collective breath each time. When I found my tumor, I knew that taking care of both breasts at the same time was absolutely the only way for me to handle my treatment. I said repeatedly, "I am doing this once."

When I asked myself that "why" Ankit talks about at the opening of this chapter—why had I gotten cancer?—one of my big answers was "stress." Mom got her diagnosis of breast cancer the year after my dad died leaving her with two teenagers who were in or going to be in college, one of whom was planning on going to med school. She also had a farm to take care of and she was a schoolteacher. My stress was autism—not only in taking care of my many patients and my own autistic daughter, but in writing a book about autism, speaking at conferences, maintaining medical practices in two different cities, traveling the world to educate as many people as I could possibly reach about autism treatment. I knew, after my diagnosis, that I would have to learn how to manage my stress in a healthier manner. I also knew that, for me as for most every other person in our harried, modern world, removing all sources of stress was just not going to be possible. I wanted to do everything that was currently medically possible to prevent a second bout of cancer in my life. I weighed this desire against my life circumstances—most notably that I had already given birth to all the children I was going to have—and made the decision to have a mastectomy to treat my cancerous breast, and a prophylactic mastectomy on my still-healthy breast.

My son's kindergarten teacher, Kristy, is one of five

sisters. She developed breast cancer when she was thirty-three years old; this happened just five years after her older sister had developed it at age thirty-one. BRCA testing was emerging on the scene when Kristy developed cancer. In addition to becoming a fierce advocate for screening, she made sure that her sisters were tested for the BRCA gene. All the sisters were tested and found that Dad had the gene—and had shared it with all five of his daughters. Each daughter was then faced with the decision about how to react to her new knowledge. Some of the sisters were already married and had children, and some of them were not—circumstances that informed their individual choices. The sisters who weren't yet married, and who hadn't yet had children, did not have prophylactic mastectomies but began a stepped-up routine to monitor their breast and ovarian health. They alternated MRI and mammography year-to-year, monitored their CA-125[1] levels, and had ovarian ultrasounds annually until they'd had children and were individually ready for prophylactic mastectomies. Their father is monitored closely for prostate, pancreatic and breast cancer as well as melanoma, all things for which he is at higher risk as a male carrier of this gene. While all the sisters have made individualized decisions about treatment or prophylactic approaches, they don't create stress for each other by arguing about their differences, but are lovingly supportive of the choices each has made.

---

1 http://www.nytimes.com/2013/05/14/opinion/my-medical-choice.html?_r=0.

tial neurological disease—and cancer. The latest studies show that DES daughters may have an increased risk of breast cancer of up to 40%.[86]

● **Arrangement of connective tissue in the breast.** A relatively new breast cancer risk factor (the first study was published in March 2011[87])—and/or a potential tool to help determine a patient's treatment and prognosis—is the way in which collagen is arranged in the connective tissue of the breast. Connective tissue, as we noted earlier in this book, is pervasive throughout our bodies, surrounding most of our organs and giving them structure; it is distinct from tissue that is specialized to perform the functions of a particular organ such as liver or kidneys, uterus or breast. Collagen, which is chemically a protein, is the main component of connective tissue. Researchers at the University of Wisconsin-Madison, School of Medicine and Public Health have discovered that the ·pattern formed by the collagen in an individual breast may be telling. That is, under a microscope, individual strands of collagen in a healthy breast look like gently curving spaghetti noodles, but near the site of a tumor the collagen becomes rigid, and looks like a clutter of pick-up-sticks. What are the implications of this discov-

---

86 http://www.cancer.gov/cancertopics/causes/des/daughters-exposed-to-des.

87 http://www.med.wisc.edu/news-events/news/ arrangement-of-connective-tissue-predicts-breast-cancer-prognosis/30720.

ery? "We think the cancer cells start to pull on the collagen and straighten it out, forming a track or highway on which the cells can migrate," says Dr. Patricia Keely, the senior author of the new study. How early in the disease process do these "highways" form? We already know that in early-stage breast cancer the collagen appears to align itself along one track and then, as the cancer becomes invasive, to realign itself. We're looking forward to ongoing studies, and what this important new discovery might be able to tell us about breast cancer risk and treatment, as well as about how it might be applied to the beneficial treatment of other types of cancer.

Risk Factors We Can Change

There are also risk factors that *can* be changed—lifestyle choices that can be either embraced or avoided in order to reduce the odds of getting the disease. Because breast cancer is a *hormonal cancer*—meaning a cancer whose growth is impacted by exposure to hormones such as estrogen and progesterone—let's discuss the risk factors that seem to involve hormone exposure first. Take note as we begin this discussion, however, that in the following section we are going to talk about hormones without making the distinction between biochemical hormones such as estrogen and chemical estrogens, known as Xenoestrogens. Xenoestrogens are not yet widely understood as a general health—and cancer—hazard, so we have decided to devote a full chapter to them in this book. (See Chapter Six.)

- **Having children.** Certainly bringing children into the world is not a decision that can be made solely on the basis of sidestepping a potential health risk, but the evidence is clear that the younger a woman is when she has children (under thirty years old) and the more children she has during her lifetime decrease slightly the risk of developing breast cancer. The reason for this is thought to be hormone-related: pregnancy reduces the amount of menstrual cycles a woman experiences over the course of a lifetime; the less menstrual cycles she experiences, the less cycle-related hormones to which she is exposed.

- **Breastfeeding.** Similarly, breastfeeding can reduce menstrual cycles, and this is thought to be related to the fact that women who have breastfed in their lifetimes have a slightly lowered risk for developing breast cancer. The caveat here is that this has been a difficult premise to study: it is believed that breastfeeding, as a significant cancer-reducing factor, has to continue over a period of time between one and a half to two years and, at least in the U.S., breastfeeding for this long is not common.

- **Oral contraceptive use.** The birth control pill became available in 1957, but it was marketed as a pill for the treatment of severe menstrual disorders; its side effect, contraception, was not widely noted until *The New York Times* ran an article, on November 21 of that year, about the debate three clergymen in Rochester, New York were initiating over that little known side effect.[88] The Pill as a cultural phenomenon was on its way. The Pill works by suppressing natural cyclical hormones through an oral dose of a small amount of synthetic estrogen and pro-gestin. This small dose of hormones causes three things to happen: the ovary is usually prevented from releasing an egg; the cervical mucus changes consistency so that a sperm has a hard time locating an egg if it is released; the lining of the uterus changes so that, should a fertilized egg find its way there, it is an inhospitable environment. It also causes various other side effects that have been fairly extensively documented through the years—from weight gain and mood changes to blurred vision, blood clots and severe headaches. It has also been implicated in a slight increase in the risk of breast cancer, though that risk appears to decline in the years after a woman stops using the pill and, after ten years of non-use, the risk seems to be the same as if she had never taken the pill at all. The warning in relation to breast cancer is clear and simple: a woman who has any other risk factors for developing breast cancer—a family history of the disease, or a benign breast condition that warrants monitoring, as

---

88 http://www.nytimes.com/2010/10/26/health/26first.html.

examples—should discuss these with her doctor before putting herself on a hormonal contraceptive.

- **Hormone replacement therapy after menopause.** There are benefits as well as risks to hormone replacement therapy: it can reduce or relieve the symptoms of menopause, such as hot flashes, night sweats, headaches and mood changes, and it can help to prevent osteoporosis, or thinning of the bones, a problem with which a full 50% of women who are over the age of fifty suffer and which is responsible for more than one and a half million bone fractures each year, so it is not a trivial consideration. The risks—as with any choice that impacts upon a woman's hormone exposure—include increased incidence of breast cancer. There are two main types of hormone therapy and each has a different impact on the significance of the risk. *Combined hormone therapy*, or *HT*, is usually prescribed for women who still have a uterus—that is, they have not had a hysterectomy—and involves both estrogen and progesterone. The progesterone is added to the mix because estrogen alone can increase the risk of uterine cancer and progesterone helps to prevent this. The increased risk of breast cancer with HT use seems to apply only to recent and current users and, five years after discontinuing its use, the risk appears to return to that of the general population. For women who no longer have a uterus, *estrogen replacement therapy*, or *ERT* (or, as it is also sometimes called, *estrogen therapy* or *ET*), which involves estrogen alone can be prescribed. The jury is still out about whether or not there is a statistically significant risk of breast cancer development with the use of ERT.[89] The good news is that a woman who has determined, after consultation with her doctor, to weigh risk factors against health benefits of HT or ERT, is not limited to "one size fits all" doses of the hormones. The doses as well as the combination can be "tweaked" to find the right balance for each individual woman, and most doctors will recommend starting with the lowest, and so least risky, dose possible.

● **Weight.** You might not immediately make the connection between your exposure to hormones and how much you weigh—and how these combined factors may contribute to the potential for breast cancer—so let's tackle this rather complicated relationship by starting with one important fact: before menopause, most of a woman's estrogen is made by her ovaries; after menopause, the ovaries stop making estrogen and most of a woman's natural estrogen supply comes from her fat tissue. What that means, in terms of the health of an individual woman, is that if she is overweight after menopause, she has a higher risk of developing breast cancer than a lean woman

---

89 The British "Million Women Study," and many other studies like this, reported a very slight increase in breast cancer risk (about 1% to 3% increase per each year of use) among women who took ET, compared to women who took the placebo.

because her body is exposed to more estrogen. But that is just one part of a complex understanding of how weight impacts on breast cancer risk. If, for example, the weight is gained as an adult, the risk for breast cancer is greater than if the woman has been overweight all of her life. Or if the woman carries the weight in her stomach area, her breast cancer risk may be greater than that of a woman who carries the weight in her thighs and hips. Or if she has high insulin levels, as is common for overweight people, then it may be the link between higher insulin levels and breast cancer—a link that has been established by medical research—that will increase her risk of the disease, rather than the increased estrogen levels being produced by excessive fat tissue. Are you African-American? Then you will be interested in the studies that show obesity may be less of a risk factor for African-American women than for other populations.[90] Are you Hispanic? Then you will take note of studies indicating that in this population the risk of breast cancer is almost doubled for overweight women.[91] But then, just when you think you understand all the possible connections between weight and breast cancer risk, you're left with the fact that some studies show that women who are overweight as *young* women have a *reduced* risk of breast cancer. With so many variables, the bottom line is that we should all try

90 http://www.cancer.gov/cancertopics/factsheet/Risk/obesity.

91 Ibid.

to achieve and maintain a healthy weight or BMI. BMI stands for body mass index, or the ratio between your weight compared to your height.[92] Except for big athletes, like football players and weight lifters who have lots of muscle, a BMI over 25 indicates that one is carrying too much body weight.

● **Diet, dietary supplements, and exercise.** There is an old-fashioned, tried-and-true formula for achieving a more ideal BMI, and it will never be replaced by any get-thin-quick scheme: diet and exercise; eating an appropriate number of wholesome calories every day and taking part in regular physical activity. In the eyes of functional medicine professionals, the foods and supplements we put into our body to create energy, and the energy we expend through exercise, are two of the most primary ways we maintain our health. In this book we think they're so important that they are worthy of whole chapters and you'll read more about them in the upcoming pages. But right now, let's take a look at what the established medical world has to say about how these factors influence breast cancer risk.

  • *Diet.* In the absence of a plethora of studies that prove a point so conclusively that the only wiggle room left would necessarily involve something smaller than a

---

92 Go here for convenient BMI Tables prepared by the Nation Institutes of Health: http://www.nhlbi.nih.gov/guidelines/obesity/bmi_tbl.htm.

BIO-IDENTICAL HORMONES

Bio-identical hormones are sometimes called "natural" hormones, so I think some attention to language is the first place to start when talking about them. "Natural" means a thing that appears in nature—and that is all it means. So when someone tells you that a food or a medicine is "natural", remind him that arsenic is as natural as the urine of a pregnant mare, which is what Premarin (which is *not* a bio-identical hormone) is made from. Bio-identical means something very specific: bio-identical hormones are hormones that are identical in molecular structure to the hormones in women's own bodies, and they interact with the other chemicals in our bodies in just the same way as the hormones our bodies produce. Of course, they are not found in this form "naturally"; they are synthesized from chemicals that are extracted from plants, gener-

sardine, the established medical community is often hard-pressed to admit that a thing works. So, while we know about the connection between, say, oxidative stress and disease, and the further connection between the antioxidants contained in fruits and vegetables and our sustained good health, the leap between staying healthy by eating fruits and vegetables and preventing or treating disease by eating fruits and vegetables is not yet complete. Most doctors now ally soy and yams. The body can't tell these bio-identical hormones from the ones that are produced by the ovaries. Indeed, a blood test of a woman who uses bio-identical hormones will reflect the estrogen supplement and the estrogen produced in her body without distinction. A blood test of a woman on a non-bio-identical hormone, on the other hand, will reflect a mix of estrogens (some of them, to use Premarin again as an example, unique to horses), steroids, and other substances.

Bio-identical hormones are FDA-approved—because they have been shown in clinical trials to reduce the chance of osteoporosis and to relieve menopausal symptoms. Controversy, however, clouds their reputation, and some of the reason for this is that some people still believe that they can only be obtained as custom formulas from compounding pharmacies[1]; this is not completely true as there are a few forms available at traditional pharmacies. As we have already said, functional medicine does not take a one-size-fits-all approach to health; custom mixture may be required if a doctor wants to prescribe medicines (hormones, in this case) in doses or combinations, or sometimes forms (powders, liquids, creams) that are not generally available.

---

[1] "Pharmacy compounding is a practice in which a licensed pharmacist combines, mixes, or alters ingredients in response to a prescription to create a medication tailored to the medical needs of an individual patient. Pharmacy compounding, if done properly, can serve an important public health need if a patient cannot be treated with an FDA-approved medication." http://www.fda.gov/drugs/Guidance-ComplianceRegulatoryInformation/PharmacyCompounding/.

advise, at the very least, a diet that emphasizes plant
sources, whole grains over refined, and a limitation on
the consumption of red and processed meats. They
will also recommend a diet that emphasizes healthy
fats and striking a very thoughtful balance between
healthy fats, protein, and carbohydrates. As we've said,
there is a definite connection between obesity and
cancer, but it is important to recognize that eating
healthy fats does not make us fat; rather, eating too
many calories without burning them off with exercise
makes us fat.

- *Exercise.* More heartening is the "official" endorse-
  ment of exercise. According to the National Cancer
  Institute, women who exercise for a minimum of
  four hours a week may reduce their risk of developing breast cancer.[93] This may have something to do
  with the fact that exercise can help to decrease hormone levels (thus lessening a woman's exposure to the
  growth effects of estrogen and progestin). But how
  much exercise, and of what kind? The American Cancer Society recommends at least half an hour of moderate to vigorous exercise five or more days a week
  for adults.[94] One study from the Women's Health

---

93 http://www.cancer.gov/cancertopics/pdq/prevention/breast/Patient/page3.

94 http://www.cancer.org/Healthy/EatHealthyGetActive/ACS-
GuidelinesonNutritionPhysicalActivityforCancerPrevention/
acs-guidelines-on-nutrition-and-physical-activity-for-cancer-prevention-intro.

Initiative of the National Institutes for Health found that women who engage in as little as 1.25 to 2.5 hours of brisk walking every week can decrease their risk of breast cancer by up to 18%.[95]

- **Alcohol.** The overuse of alcohol increases one's risk of breast cancer; that fact has been demonstrated to the satisfaction of the establishment.[96] And, more specifically, the risk of hormone-receptor-positive invasive breast cancer may be especially acute due to the abusive effects of alcohol. Now, as both of your authors like a glass of wine now and again, we take care to report that it is in higher quantity that alcohol can cause its damage: women who have one or fewer drinks per day do not seem to experience risk greater than non-drinkers do; those who drink one to two, or more than two glasses per day, however, could experience a significant increase in risk.

- **Antiperspirants and other environmental chemicals.** For years there has been speculation that antiperspirants—or, more specifically, the *parabens* in antiperspirants, which are a class of chemicals that are widely used in the cosmetic as well as pharmaceutical industries as preservatives—caused cancer. The speculation was bolstered by a small study in 2004 that found a link between

---

95 http://www.ncbi.nlm.nih.gov/pubmed/12966124.

96 http://www.ncbi.nlm.nih.gov/pubmed/3104648.

underarm shaving, the parabens in antiperspirants and cancer: it was theorized that the parabens, which do have estrogen-like properties, albeit weak ones, entered the body through nicks and other irritations caused by shaving and caused cancer.[97] While we can't give weight to this specific speculation about parabens as an *isolated* contributor to breast cancer development, what we can do is speak to the larger issue: the cumulative effects of environmental assault that we all face daily—e.g., paraben preservatives in cosmetics and medicines we put on our skin, carcinogenic chemicals in plastic residues and pesticides and cleaning solvents we get on our hands, particulate matter and heavy metals in the air we breathe and the water we drink. We know that these substances change our cellular activity, weaken our cellular structure, and damage our DNA—and, you will recall, damaged DNA is what leads to cancer. It is not likely, however, that exposure to one chemical agent (a paraben) placed in one particular area (under the arm, near the breast) can be held responsible for causing one disease; it is, rather, the whole host of environmental toxins to which we are regularly exposed that, combined, manifest as diseases like breast cancer.[98] The most reasonable approach is

---

97 http://terranaturals.com/pdf/mcgrath_full.pdf.

98 "Environmental Risks and Breast Cancer" is a collaborative effort of the faculty, students and technical professionals at Vassar College and a substantial reference for learning more about the role of everyday chemicals and other toxins in the

not to be afraid of your antiperspirant, specifically, but to make the replacement of your antiperspirant with a deodorant stone or crystal only one of the beneficial life-style choices you make in opting for breast health.

- **Bras.** Does underwear cause cancer? Bras, and in particular the underwire sort, have come under such suspicion that the bra-cancer link has become a bit of an urban legend. The theory is that bras cause breast cancer by obstructing the flow of lymph fluids draining from the breast area. No solid proof exists at this time that links bras with breast cancer, though the speculation is that women with smaller breasts—that is, women with less dense breast tissue and, so, a lesser risk of developing breast cancer—tend to be the women who go without bras and this may account for any anecdotal evidence that there is a correlation between underwear and disease.

- **Induced or spontaneous abortions.** There have been really a glut of major studies conducted worldwide on the possible link between abortion and breast cancer, and their findings are consistent: neither spontaneous abortion (miscarriage) nor induced abortion (the medical termination of a pregnancy) nor stillbirths (which are, medically, considered a type of abortion) can be linked to

---

development of breast cancer: http://erbc.vassar.edu/erbc/environmentalrisks/out-sidethehome/metals/index.html.

breast cancer. The first such study was conducted in Denmark in 1997,[99] a study we highlight as just one of many for the sake of space limitations.

- **Breast implants.** Researchers have found no direct link between breast implants and breast cancer.[100] What is understood is that silicone implants can cause scar tissue to form in the breast, and this can make it more difficult to interpret standard mammograms. Women with breast implants should make sure they inform their radiologist of their implants during their annual mammogram so that he or she can take additional x-rays, called *implant displacement views*, which assure the breast is examined more completely.

- **Smoking/second-hand smoke.** Smoking is bad for your health. There is simply no dispute on that issue. But does smoking, or exposure to second-hand smoke, cause breast cancer? Researchers have found no direct link and even the 2006 U.S. Surgeon General's report, *The Health Consequences of Involuntary Exposure to Tobacco Smoke*, went only so far as to say that there is "suggestive but not sufficient" evidence of a link. Nicotine, however, the addictive alkaloid in the nightshade plant tobacco, is a chemical, and it should be categorized right at the top of

---

99 http://www.nejm.org/doi/full/10.1056/NEJM199701093360201.

100 http://www.cancer.gov/newscenter/pressreleases/2000/siliconebreast.

environmental chemicals that alter cell activity and structure, and damage DNA, whether we inhale it directly or involuntarily.

● **Night work.** As we have mentioned before, working overnight—as many nurses do, for instance—has been shown to cause a slight increase in the risk of breast cancer.[101] Indeed, in some countries this finding is understood in such a mainstream and compassionate way that employers have begun compensating their workers who develop breast cancer after a number of years working the night shift.[102]

It is, of course, not possible to predict with any certainty exactly which woman is going to be diagnosed with breast cancer and which one is not. "Why me?"—as my patients so clearly understand—is as valid a question as "Why *not* me?" But the value of knowing the risk factors that can cause or contribute to a diagnosis of breast cancer is in being able to act on them—to change the things we can so we increase our odds of surviving breast cancer, or even of avoiding it altogether.

---

101 http://www.ncbi.nlm.nih.gov/pubmed/16357603.

102 http://articles.cnn.com/2009-03-16/health/cancer.
nightwork_1_breast-cancer-night-work-shifts?_s=PM:HEALTH.

6

Nix the Xenoestrogens

What do your favorite cozy chair, your
shampoo and the chicken you're going to
cook for dinner tonight have in common?

Julie

That might sound like a strange riddle right now, but by the end of this chapter you'll understand the connection between these three dissimilar items—and the connection might well alarm you, though we hope you'll respond to any apprehension in the same way we hope you've already responded to knowing that tobacco is bad for you: by quitting smoking and/or avoiding second-hand smoke. Knowledge is, of course, power and the intent of this chapter is to give you the power to avoid one particular risk factor for breast cancer that is so insidious we believe it deserves its own chapter in order to cover it in the depth and detail it warrants. That risk factor is *Xenoestrogens*.

What the heck are xenoestrogens? Simply put, they are chemicals that are not naturally found in the human body but that mimic the human biochemical estrogen. Bubble bath is a fun way to illustrate exactly what I mean. I love bubble baths. I have loved them since I was a little girl. Back then Mom used to keep a big pink box of Mr. Bubble near the tub and I would add liberal amounts to the warm running water to make mountains of bubbles. Once in a while—either because

I had been too liberal with the pink powder or Mom simply forgot to stock up—I would find myself ready for my evening bath with no Mr. Bubble in sight so I would head out to the kitchen and swipe the bottle of dishwashing liquid from under the sink. Now, dishwashing liquid belongs in the kitchen, not the bathtub, but in a pinch it made lots and lots of perfectly acceptable bubbles.

Similarly, though xenoestrogens do not belong in the human body, once they get inside of us the body thinks they are a perfectly acceptable substitute for biochemical estrogen and they do a bang-up job of triggering the same cellular reactions as our own natural estrogen. Unfortunately, while substituting a squirt of Joy for a sprinkle of Mr. Bubble in my youthful tub was harmless in intention, xenoestrogens can be dangerous.

As we have already discussed, breast cancer is most often a hormonal cancer, meaning that it is affected by exposure to hormones. Hormones are chemicals produced in glands such as the thyroid, ovaries and testicles that act as messengers, sending out signals that affect the growth, function and/or metabolism of cells in other parts of the body. In the popular culture we most often associate hormones with sexual arousal, or lack thereof, particularly in the context of different life phases—it is conventional wisdom that teenagers have lusty, raging hormones; mood swings that can be associated with PMS or menopause are readily chalked up to hormonal imbalance. In truth, however, hormones play a much broader role in the biochemical cascade that occurs in every single one of the estimated ten trillion cells in our body every single second of every single day. Hormones help to regulate our metabolisms, they help to prepare our bodies to cope with stress (particularly impacting our fight-or-flight response), and they control our reproductive cycles as well as our hunger cravings. Hormones also help to activate or inhibit the function of our immune systems and our nervous systems—an imbalance of hormonal activity in the body has a 360-degree ripple effect on how we can live our lives; when you mess with hormone levels it is not just one thing—a mood swing, a lack of interest in or a preoccupation with sex—that results. In fact, as science learns more about these amazingly versatile and powerful molecules, we scientists are beginning to substitute the word neuro-immuno-endocrine modulators for the word hormone. It's the scientists' way of reminding ourselves of how complex and multifaceted these chemical messengers truly are: hormones have a global impact on our body's function.

Let us zero in, however, on one more of the specific roles that hormones play in our internal, biochemical lives—and that is to initiate or suppress *apoptosis*, also called programmed cell death. Programmed cell death is a normal, necessary process of the human body, though the life span of a cell depends on its particular function—a cell that makes up our stomach lining lives for about two days while a red blood cell can live about four months. A skin cell lives for two to four weeks, a bone cell for twenty-five to thirty years. A category of white blood cell called granulocytes can live for as little as ten hours but a brain cell can live for as long as you do. When the hormonal balance is disrupted, however, it can, in turn, disrupt the process of apoptosis, playing havoc with the life cycles of the cells. Too much apoptosis can lead to *atrophy*, which is a partial or even complete wasting away of the body, whereas an insufficient amount of programmed cell death can result in an uncontrolled proliferation of cells—and cancer, by definition, is a process of unregulated cell growth.

The most common form of cancer for women is breast cancer, and the most common form of cancer for men is prostate cancer; could it be simply coincidence that both of these are hormone-modulated diseases? I don't think so. The formula is simple and direct: increase a person's exposure to hormones to levels greater than her body needs and you increase her risk for developing cancer. Xenoestrogens are, if you will, "extra-hormonal." The danger with exposure to extra, environmental hormones is that when they get inside of us the body becomes confused, it doesn't know what it is supposed to be doing. For example, for centuries the onset of female puberty began when a girl reached fifteen or sixteen years of age; since the onset of "innovations" such as industrial dairy farming that filled the marketplace with milk from hormone-laden cows, cases of girls as young as eight years old developing breasts are really not that uncommon now. Can the American obesity epidemic be blamed entirely on the proliferation of fast-food outlets, or does the fact that hormones—and the extra xenoestrogens we are all exposed to on a daily basis—impact cellular metabolism have something to do with why so many of us are fat? Unpopular as this next question might be, it must be asked: *Can our reliance on hormonal forms of birth control, such as the pill, during much of the reproductive years of so many young women, or therapies such as hormone replacement therapy (HRT) during menopause, help to explain the increase in the incidence of breast cancer among women?*

How long have we known about this formula, this connection between hormones and cancer? In 1896, a Scottish surgeon named George Beatson published a study concerning three of his patients whose breast cancer had responded favorably to the removal of their ovaries. This was science's first hint that cancer growth was impacted by hormones. Since 1937, with the invention of a chemical called diethylstillboestrol that slowed tumor activity, estrogen-blockers such as tamoxifen and other hormone-based therapies such as cortisone, have been used in cancer treatment.

We'll go into such hormone therapies in relation to the treatment of breast cancer later in this book, of course; right now let's stay focused on the role of hormones in causing cancer in the first place and ask the next logical questions: *How long have we known that both naturally occurring hormones as well as xenoestrogens can contribute to the development of cancer? How long have we known about the link between xenoestrogens and breast cancer?* Way back in 1993, the National Institutes of Health conducted a study centered on xenoestrogens as a preventable cause of breast cancer.[103] What they knew going into the study was that then-currently established risk factors for breast cancer could not explain the puzzling rise in incidence of the disease,[104] and that improved methods of detection could not fully explain the increase in cases that were being diagnosed. They wondered: "Could environmental chemicals that increase estrogen exposure by functioning as xenoestrogens explain some of the increases in breast cancer?"[105] They also wondered, in the same study, if exposure to xenoestrogens could explain the increases in other hormonally-directed biological functions—things such as incidences of reduced sperm count and increases in cases of testicular cancer that had also risen throughout the previous decades. These were good questions—indeed, these were *great* questions!—but unfortunately the study concluded on a tremendously weak note: "*If* [italics mine] xenoestrogens do play a role in breast cancer, reductions in exposure will provide an opportunity for primary prevention of this growing disease."

Since 1993, of course, many, many more studies have been conducted around these questions. Most of them are still equivocal, if not downright obtuse, about the connection between xenoestrogens and the rise in rates of hormonally-impacted disease—as an example: "The occurrence of such

---

103 *http://www.ncbi.nlm.nih.gov/pmc/articles/PMC1519851/.*

104 A sustained 1% annual increase in breast cancer mortality had been occurring since the 1940s. *http://www.ncbi.nlm.nih.gov/pmc/articles/PMC1519851/.*

105 Ibid.

converging transcriptional programs reinforces the hypothesis that multiple xenoestrogenic contaminants, of natural or anthropogenic origin, may act in conjunction with the endogenous hormone to induce additive effects in target tissues."[106] There is still a need for greater clarity around this issue, so let me present this in a way that is perfectly understandable.

Suppose you walk into your living room and click the remote control to turn on your TV, but the TV screen remains blank. Then suppose that, immediately, your eye moves to the wall socket and you see that the TV is unplugged—at least, being sometimes excessively practical, the wall socket would be the first place my eye would go. Now, seeing that the TV is unplugged, you could still, certainly, stand in front of the blank screen hypothesizing the many reasons why the TV was not working. You could wonder if the cable company was doing some work in your neighborhood that affected its delivery, or you could decide the power company had a line down and you were suffering an outage, or you could fret that your TV set itself was broken. Or, you could try plugging the set back into the wall and, in 99.99999% of cases, this would mean that in about ten seconds you'd be sitting down in front of it to watch your favorite show.

One of my favorite sayings is, "If it looks like a duck, and quacks like a duck and waddles like a duck, it is probably a duck." And I know a duck when I see one. In our example—and if you will allow me to strangle a metaphor—that

---

106 *http://carcin.oxfordjournals.org/content/27/8/1567.short.*

unplugged TV cord is the duck. If a young patient walks into my office with a new and unexplained rash on his tummy, the first thing I'm going to ask Mom about is her laundry detergent and soap—and in 99.99999% of the cases we're going to find out that the young patient is having an allergic reaction to something as innocuous as the new laundry detergent that happened to be on sale at the supermarket last week. The laundry detergent is the duck. In the case of xenoestrogens and their link to rising rates of breast cancer, I can clearly see the duck even if research scientists are as yet very cautious about what they call that animal they've been studying.

Now, that doesn't mean that the researchers who are conducting what continue to be important studies on this link are missing the forest for the trees. What it does mean is that there is a critical dependency, as well as critical difference, between the research scientists and the clinicians, like me, who use the results of research in treating real, live patients every day of the week. This difference gets at the heart of one of my favorite points when debating therapeutic interventions with researchers and academicians—the question of evidence-based medicine. Those who work in the medical field who are involved in research trials very often insist that the only treatment approaches of value are those that have been "proven" with a double-blind, placebo-controlled trial. But we can forget too easily that evidence-based medicine also takes into account the cumulative clinical experience of practitioners. In fact, the questions that researchers strive to answer are formulated, in most cases indirectly, by the patients we clinicians treat—over the decades, more and more patients who turn out to have breast cancer have been walking into our offices, so our brilliant researchers walk into their labs to try to find out why more women are getting the disease. The researchers may or may not find a definitive answer or—more commonly—find what *could be* a definitive answer, but then fail to come to any sort of consensus about how their findings can or should be used in practice. This lack of consensus can lead to different clinicians recommending different approaches to disease treatment; if the opinions of the research scientists diverge too greatly, the lack of consensus can lead to controversy.

For example, let's not forget—evidence that cigarettes caused cancer began to pile up in the 1920s,[107] but as late as 1949 four out of five doctors smoked Camels.[108] For many observant clinicians of the time, cigarettes were indeed a duck, but researchers did not clearly and unanimously agree with them and so, for decades, while doctors could offer patients the opinion that quitting smoking would be beneficial for their health, they had no scientific consensus to solidly support that position. What they had, instead of scientific consensus—and in spite of, I might add, loud and liberal lobbying from the tobacco industry—was evidence that walked into their offices every day on its own two feet: patients who were healthier when they did not smoke or whose health improved when they gave it up.

---

107 *http://cebp.aacrjournals.org/content/16/6/1070.full.*

108 *http://www.youtube.com/watch?v=gCMzjJjuxQI.*

Like those prescient physicians of the 1940s and 1950s who were unwilling to wait for undisputable scientific consensus surrounding the dangers of smoking before they advised their patients to quit—and unwilling to wait either for the cultural consensus that came even decades after that—I am unwilling to wait to sound the alarm about xenoestrogens. Given the semi-direct sources of xenoestrogens to which we are commonly exposed—say, bovine antibiotics in the milk most of us drink—and the direct xenoestrogens that end up in our bodies—such as birth control pills—we shouldn't be surprised that more and more of us are developing cancer.

The good news is that avoiding many of the worst sources of xenoestrogens is often not complex—and solutions to the problem of xenoestrogen exposure are not, in context, really that costly.

What do I mean by those seemingly sneaky words, "in context"? Well, the other morning I dropped my car off for service. It needed a routine oil change, and the driver's side windshield wiper wasn't functioning properly—wasn't effectively clearing raindrops from my field of vision—so I wanted to have the wiper blades replaced. I ended up spending about $93 for this service, not an insignificant amount of money for most middle-class families like mine. I could have, I suppose, saved the money, put off the oil change or scrunched down in the driver's seat in the car when it rained so I could see out the portion of the window that the wiper actually still cleared. But had I done those things I would have risked causing damage to the car's engine—and, worse, I would have risked causing an accident if I couldn't see the road properly in a rainstorm. The cost—both in dollars and cents as well as potential risk to life—could have been exponentially greater had I put off caring for my car.

The problem—the *irony*—is that, for most people, taking preventative care of our cars takes priority over taking preventative caring for our bodies. Perhaps that's because we experience the results of a neglected car so much more immediately, and visually, than we experience the results of neglected health. We can actually see that a defective wiper blade is making it difficult to see out a windshield; we can't see or hear or feel the damage a xenoestrogen is causing inside of our bodies until, often, the damage is so great we need to seek medical treatment. We do, however, possess the knowledge to take as good care of ourselves as we take of our cars—and if we use this knowledge we can help to prevent disease. An ounce of prevention is still worth a pound of cure; in context, that ounce of prevention still costs a lot less than the pound—and the pain—of cure.

All right, then; I've convinced you about the benefits of prevention! How do you avoid xenoestrogens and prevent the damage they can cause?[109]

---

109 You can go here to download an Excel spreadsheet that contains a comprehensive list of currently-known estrogenic chemical ingredients. *http://www.endocrinedisruption.com/endocrine.TEDXList.overview.php*. This list, however, could

Xenoestrogens find their way into your body in three different ways: orally, in the foods you eat and the medications and supplements you take; through your skin, or transdermally; and in the air you breathe.

The single most important first step to take in cleaning up your body and ridding it of the accumulated and on-going effects of xenoestrogens is to clean up what you eat. This clean-up includes switching, as the family budget will allow, to buying and eating organic foods. If you are on a tight budget—and who among us doesn't deal with a budget of some tension these days—refer to the "Dirty Dozen" list in Chapter Four for the twelve most important fruits and vegetables to buy organic. Organic produce is fruits and vegetables that have been grown without the use of such things as chemical or petroleum-based fertilizers, herbicides, pesticides and fungicides. Peel non-organic produce before you eat it. Do your best to either eat less meat or to buy meats that come from animals that haven't been dosed with antibiotics to assist the process of fattening them up; if you do eat non-organic meat, avoid eating the fat as this is where the bulk of accumulated xenoestrogens are stored in animals. If you still drink cow's milk, organic brands that, again, don't come from cows that have been dosed with antibiotics to increase production, are your best bet. Additionally, try to avoid canned goods; convenient

---

prove daunting; I recommend a more "common sense" approach, as outlined in the balance of this chapter.

as these can be, the cans have nearly always been lined with the xenoestrogen, Bisphenol A.

It's worth mentioning at this juncture that soy is a hot topic in terms of estrogen. And as we think about soy, it becomes more obvious why there appears to be disagreement. Remember that soy is never available to your body as just soy. It's soy that may or may not be a genetically modified organism, or GMO. GMOs are modified by seed production companies in an attempt to make super plants that don't succumb to pestilence, drought, or other natural variables as they grow. Soy may or may not be organic; you may get a few other chemicals with your soy when you eat it. Soy then has to be digested in your gut, travel past an immune system that is probably, since you are reading this book, upside down and confused enough to be allowing cancer to grow, metabolized by your liver, and then utilized by your particular body and your particular hormone receptors. There are studies that talk about how soy increases estrogen—and there are studies that say soy increases only the "good" estrogen. We also know that soy is a source of isoflavones that can lower your estrogen levels. How soy influences estrogen depends in part on how much of which kinds of estrogen you already have floating around in your body. Which, in the end, leaves us standing at the dairy section in the grocery store, with our hand moving back and forth from the soy yogurt to the coconut yogurt, completely confused as to what to do. Current consensus in my functional medicine world is that organic, non-GMO soy is probably not a significant problem in terms of having estrogenic properties, whereas GMO conventionally-grown soy is probably a pro-estrogenic food that should be avoided.[110] I, personally, don't eat a lot of soy. I choose the coconut yogurt, but allow myself the soy-derived cream cheese and sour cream that I love, and use a carefully isolated isoflavone to keep estrogen lower in my post-cancer life.

Next, clean up your cleaning products, garden products, and personal care products. Use up the chemical-laden products under your kitchen sink and replace them with chemical-free and biodegradable brands like Seventh Generation, Green the Cleaning, Simple Green, and Green Works, which is actually a Clorox product. Switch from chemically-based pesticides and fertilizers to natural products for your lawn and garden and, if you use a lawn service, choose one that doesn't spray, as most lawn care sprays are loaded with xenoestrogens. More and more, there are organic or, at least, "natural" choices if you ask your lawn service company to provide them, and there are actually organic lawn service companies popping up all over suburbia these days as more and more people not only express but act on concerns about living with too many chemicals. Choose soaps, shampoos, deodorants, toothpastes and other personal care products that don't include estrogenic ingredients and other toxic chemicals such as parabens and

---

110 Presented at the Functional Medicine AFMCP Course in Portland, Oregon, September 2010.

stearalkonium chloride in their make-up. Avoid plug-in air fresheners since you inhale the formaldehyde in their formulas along with their chemically-pleasant scents. Choose insect repellants made with all-natural ingredients—and choose sun blocks (which are mineral-based, like zinc oxide, and sit on the surface of your skin) rather than sunscreens (that are chemical-based and need to be absorbed by the skin in order to be effective) to protect yourself from burning during your day at the beach.

Pay attention to the sorts of paper products you purchase—choose chlorine-free, unbleached paper towels, napkins, toilet paper and coffee filters. A study by the Environmental Protection Agency (EPA) has found that exposure to dioxins from the use of bleached coffee filters is, of itself, enough to exceed the lifetime "acceptable" limit of dioxin ingestion—though I am hard-pressed to think of a level that could be thought of as "acceptable". Importantly, make sure your tampons and menstrual pads are chlorine-free, too.

Install a tap filter in your home for water; "city water" can contain chlorine, fluoride, and other industrial and agricultural chemicals.

Use plastics as little as humanly possible, especially for food consumption and storage; plastics release a chemical known as bisphenol A (BPA) that leeches from the plastic and into the food, especially under heat. Use ceramic or glass containers as often as you can to store food, and to drink and eat from. Never, never, never microwave food that is placed in plastic containers or that is covered with a plastic wrap; if you're, say, on a hike, and drinking water out of a plastic bottle, don't allow the bottle to heat up from the sun. Don't refill plastic water bottles and don't freeze in them and later drink the water.

Choose family-planning methods that are not hormonally-based—barrier methods such as diaphragms and condoms can be good alternatives but be sure to read the labels on condoms and diaphragm gels as lubricants and gels can contain estrogenic chemicals.

If you're lucky enough to be in a position to redecorate your home, avoid synthetic carpets, particle-board and some faux wood products as they can contain or may have been manufactured with products containing estrogenic disruptors and can leech or "off-gas" noxious gases. Choose furniture and fabrics that have not been manufactured using various chemical processes as these too can leech noxious fumes for years. In order to offset leeching that may already be occurring in your home, there are several popular plants that absorb toxins from the air as they grow; these include many vining plants like English Ivy and philodendrons, ferns like sword and Boston species, many palms such as bamboo palm and dwarf date palm, and some flowering plants, such as blue daisies. Consider adding a few of them to your décor if you have even a slightly green thumb.

Wear protective gloves if you find yourself unable to avoid working with solvents, glues, cleaning solutions or other cleaning or hobby products that contain xenoestrogens, and be sure to ventilate appropriately while you are using them.

Finally, though it is difficult to avoid completely in our modern, busy world the noxious fumes that come from office equipment such as copiers and printers, from the gas pump or the exhaust fumes of other cars on the road, or from the fossil-fuel-burning power plants that supply so much of our electricity, try to condition yourself to become aware of them so you can decrease your exposure as much as is possible. At the office, have that conversation about last night's episode of *Glee* at your desk rather than in the copy room. Ask yourself if you could maybe walk to the post office or convenience store instead of driving. If the luxury of moving even further away from your town or region's power plant is within your grasp, do it.

As I said, cleaning up the estrogenic toxins in your environment can seem daunting. A common sense, step-by-step approach—doing one thing today and another next week and making a third healthy lifestyle choice next month—is better than allowing yourself to be overwhelmed or discouraged by trying to do too much all at once. At my house, we focused on getting organic gradually, as the budget would allow. First the dirty dozen foods were cleaned up, and then we worked on other foods. It took a little while until I could focus on the toothpastes, shampoos, and window cleaners. I had to remind myself that the tortoise eventually beat the hare in that storied race from childhood—even a little cleanup is certainly better than doing nothing! And though you may not immediately see or hear or even feel the benefits of your efforts, by reminding yourself that you are doing something infinitely positive for your family, you can experience the psychic lift in each small incremental change that can keep you moving forward toward a healthier, more chemical-free life. I promise you, eventually, you *will* feel the rewards of your efforts—and it will feel *good*!

7

Your Lab Reports— Simplified

You're always just a little less afraid of things
you know than of things you don't know.

Ankit

When my wife and I head into the kitchen to make dinner at the end of the day, we're pretty sure that whatever we cook is going to end up edible. In fact, unless we're trying out some exotic new recipe, we don't give eventual edibility a single thought—we're competent home cooks, we can roast and steam and boil and sauté with the best of them, and we have a working knowledge of what herbs and spices will complement which meats and vegetables; we know the basics. When we do decide we want to try that exotic new dish, we're not intimidated by new techniques or ingredients because we have a grasp of fundamentals that allows us to learn in a way that is not only efficient, but fun.

There are, however, certain other chores necessary to the smooth functioning of the household that neither one of us would approach with confidence—changing the oil in our car, installing the plumbing in the new half bath, hanging the wallpaper in the baby's room. These are common tasks that some people might have the inclination or talent to do themselves, but given our areas of interest and experience, we choose to call in a professional when they need to be done.

Similarly, each professional more often than not has a defined area of expertise—you don't go to a body shop, for example, to have your oil changed. When you need legal advice about your tax return, you don't go to an attorney who specializes in trial law. When you're making your annual mammogram appointment, you don't call your dermatologist.

Yet, when a woman is diagnosed with breast cancer, she has no choice but to become a medical expert, with a specialty in breast cancer, and to do it *fast*. This reality is stressful and unfair—but not impossible.

Typically there is a period of about one month between the time a woman is diagnosed with breast cancer and the time that her treatment begins. A lot has to happen in this relatively brief span of time. These things range from the highly personal and emotionally nuanced—for example, shifting one's whole mental and emotional landscape to include the cancer diagnosis—to the highly scientific and biochemically subtle. In one month—while in the midst of an illness that potentially can involve the loss of her breasts, the ordeal of chemotherapy and the upheaval of family and work routines, not to mention the dynamics surrounding them—a woman has to, essentially, put herself through a rigorous, often self-taught medical residency, learning about the disease and the treatments that are available for *her particular manifestation of the disease.* Then she must make decisions that will not only save her life, but that she will live with for the rest of her life. It's a tall order.

Part of the mission that Julie and I set for ourselves when we decided to write this book together was to make the "residency program" that each breast cancer patient is forced into upon her diagnosis a little less rigorous. To provide, in one handy place, the basic information that every newly diagnosed breast cancer patient should have right up front, so that she has the best chance of becoming her own best advocate—of making informed choices about treatment options that are right for *her* and her lifestyle, and then making any necessary changes in that lifestyle that will help keep her healthy after she has beaten the cancer.

So, where do you start, in the midst of a difficult emotional landscape, to digest, and then act on, the information *you'll* need? What's the first step? We suggest it is taking control of your *pathology report*. Why this as a first step? Let's back up a little and I'll explain.

No two women experience breast cancer in exactly the same way. No treatment, no procedure is right for every patient. Where the cancer is located, its size and appearance, how quickly it grows and if or how far it has spread, if it is affected by hormones—these are some of the factors that will determine each woman's unique path to recovery. Moreover, if mastectomy is recommended as part of the treatment process, the reconstruction options that are available and appropriate will depend, in large part, on these factors as well. You find out what these factors are through *lab tests*. All your lab tests, taken together, comprise your pathology report.

There are a wide variety of lab tests that are available to help a doctor and her patient make informed breast cancer treatment decisions. But not all of the lab tests that are available to assist in your diagnosis are routine—your doctor may order some tests, but not others, depending on the information she needs to assess your particular cancer experience. And it also isn't routine that all of these tests are ordered at the same time—for example, some of the tests are done at the time of the initial biopsy when suspect tissue and nearby tissues are tested, and others are done after surgery. The results of some lab tests will be available mere days after the tests are performed; others can take several weeks. Given all of these variables, taking control of your own pathology report is necessary to become a proactive, informed, *empowered* patient. One of my patients once told me that, at the start of her cancer treatment, she had felt as if she'd lost the ability to manage her life. Too much information was coming at her too quickly, and she was frankly too tired and emotionally distracted to process it. The organization and interpretation of her lab reports, however, was one aspect of cancer that she *could* control. Claiming this sort of control for yourself can help you to become confident and assertive in determining your own singular path to recovery.

What follows is a detailed breakdown of all of the different, individual reports that can comprise that larger entity, a conventional pathology report. I caution you to understand that in this book Julie and I are being comprehensive: your pathology report may or may not include each item in the breakdown below. If you have a question about what is or is not included in your personal pathology report, ask your doctor for clarification.

Non-invasive or Invasive Breast Cancer

As we have discussed in previous chapters, most often breast cancer begins in the cells of the lobules, which are the milk-producing glands, or in the ducts, which are the passageways through which milk drains from the lobules to the nipple. One of the first things you and your doctor are going to want to know is whether or not the cancer has spread outside the lobules or ducts where it originated. If it has not spread from the area of the breast where it originated, it is known as non-invasive cancer; if it has spread from the area of origin, it is called invasive cancer.

Non-invasive cancers are also referred to as pre-cancers or carcinoma *in situ*, which means, literally, *in the same place*: in this type of cancer, the cancer cells have stayed in their place of origin; they have not spread to other breast tissue outside the lobules or the ducts, and neither have they spread outside the breast. Once your doctor has determined that your cancer is non-invasive, he will further refine the classification as either DCIS or LCIS.

DCIS, or Ductal Carcinoma In Situ, is a non-invasive type of cancer that stays put in the milk duct—or, at least, stays put *temporarily*. DCIS is also considered a precancerous lesion, which means that, if undetected or untreated, it will likely develop into an invasive cancer.

LCIS, or Lobular Carcinoma In Situ, is not a true cancer. It is, rather, an over abundance of abnormal cells that grow inside the lobule. An LCIS is considered precancerous: a warning sign for an increased risk of developing invasive breast cancer, *in either breast, not only the one in which it is discovered.*

Invasive cancers, on the other hand, *do* grow into the healthy tissue that surrounds them—the membrane that lines a duct or a lobule—thus *invading* or *infiltrating* the normal tissue. The cancer cells can then, in this case, travel to other parts of the body, such as the lymph nodes.

Unfortunately, most breast cancers are invasive. The most common type of breast cancer, in fact, is IDC, or Invasive Ductal Carcinoma, which begins in the milk duct but spreads into the surrounding healthy tissue inside the breast.

Less common are some of the subtypes of Invasive Ductal Carcinoma, such as *tubular, medullary, mucinous, papillary,* and *cribriform* carcinomas. These less-than-common words are, simply, descriptions of the way the cancer cells appear when they are looked at under a microscope. Cells with these types of appearance behave differently than do the cells of common invasive ductal carcinomas, and their behavior gives your doctor clues to how they may respond to treatment.

ILC, or Invasive Lobular Carcinoma, begins in the lobule but spreads to the tissue inside the breast that surrounds the site of origin.

Even less common—indeed, in rare cases—breast cancer begins not in the ducts or the lobules, but in the connective tissue, or stroma, of the breast: in the muscle or fat tissue, or in blood vessels. When the cancer begins in connective tissue, it is called *sarcoma. Phyllodes tumors* are an example of one such sarcoma; they are rare, and rarely cancerous, though they do grow quickly, and in a leaf-like pattern. *Angiosarcoma*, another example, are cancers that originate in the walls of the blood or lymphatic vessels; because of their location—within the body's 'transport' system—such cancers can spread rapidly.

Other terms you will want to know as you and your doctor discuss this classification of your cancer are:

● **Inflammatory Breast Cancer** is a fast growing cancer that starts not with a distinct lump but with a swelling of the breast or reddening of the breast skin. Typical features can also include localized warmth in the breast, and the discovery of cancer cells in the armpit, or axillary, lymph nodes, or breast skin.

● **Paget's Disease of the Nipple** is a very rare form of breast cancer in which the cancerous cells are located in or around the nipple.

● **Recurrent Breast Cancer** is cancer that has returned after a previous treatment.

● **Metastatic Breast Cancer** is cancer that has spread outside of the breast, to other parts of the body.

● **Cancer that is *both Invasive and Non-Invasive*** is, just as you would guess, a cancer that has grown, in part, outside of the site of origin and, in part, stayed put inside the lobule or duct in which it originally formed. When this sort of cancer occurs, it is treated as invasive. DCIS that has just begun to spread (i.e. microinvasion) is an example of this phenomenon.

- **Mixed Tumor** refers to a cancer that contains a mixture of ductal cells and lobular cells. This sort of cancer is usually treated as a ductal, and can be referred to by a variety of names, such as *invasive mammary breast cancer* and *infiltrating mammary carcinoma*.

- **Multifocal** breast cancer is a cancer in which there is more than one tumor in the breast, but all of the tumors that exist have grown from one original tumor, and all of the tumors are located in the same section or part of the breast.

- **Multicentric** breast cancer is a cancer in which there is more than one tumor in the breast, but all of the tumors have formed independently of each other; in this case, the tumors are frequently in different sections or parts of the breast.

Rate of Cell Growth

Cancer cells grow in a simple, straightforward way—cell division. This means that one wayward cell divides itself and becomes two wayward cells; those two cells then divide and become four; the four divide and become eight, and so on. But how *fast* do they divide? It is estimated that it can take up to two months for each division to be complete—and that it can take up to thirty divisions for the mass of cancer cells this division creates to be detected by hand, by even the most experienced doctor. This little piece of data underpins yet again the importance of regular mammograms: mammograms can detect a mass of cancer cells when it is so small that it may need to grow for up to a full year more before it can be detected in a clinical breast examination.

What 'rate of cell growth' means in terms of your pathology report is not how fast the cells are dividing, but what portion of the cancer cells are dividing and forming new cancer cells—what proportion of the tumor is engaged in growth. A higher proportion of dividing cells implies that it is likely the cancer is a more aggressive (faster growing) type; a lower proportion means, of course, just the opposite: that the cancer is a slower, less aggressive type. It is worth noting here that another way we doctors talk about this rate of growth is 'differentiation'. A poorly differentiated tumor is usually growing very quickly, and is said to be more aggressive. While this sounds like bad news, the good news is that these types of tumors very often respond beautifully (if such a thing is possible) to chemotherapy. On the other hand, you can think of well-differentiated tumors as generally fairly synonymous with less aggressive, more slowly growing cancer. 'Slower growing' is intuitively better, but well differentiated also means that the tumor cells look more like healthy tissue under the microscope and, as a result, it can be harder to target those types of tumors with chemotherapy without damaging a lot of healthy cells, too.

There are a number of tests than can measure the rate of cell growth, including the *S-phase fraction* and the *Ki-67*.

- **S-phase fraction.** 'S-phase' is shorthand for the term 'synthesis phase,' a process that happens in one cell immediately before it divides into two cells. The 'S-phase fraction' is a test that can tell you what fraction, or percentage, of the cells in a sample of tissue are in the process of copying their genetic information in anticipation of imminent division. A score of less than 6% is low, 6 to 10% intermediate, and 10% or over is high. The higher the S-phase fraction indicates a higher growth rate for your cancer.

- **Ki-67.** This test involves a staining process that can measure the percentage of the cells in a tumor that are positive for K-67, a protein that increases in a cell as it prepares to divide into two cells. If over 20% of the cells test positive for Ki-67, the cells are dividing rapidly; a result of 10 to 20% is intermediate, and less than 10% is low.

Keep in mind that while both these tests may provide you and your doctor with helpful information, experts don't always agree on how best to utilize the results for the purposes of treatment decisions because the results are not universally reliable. It is not routine, therefore, for doctors to order these tests as part of a standard pathology report. (Note, however, that if you and your doctor decide to include genomic assays, which we will talk about in just a few pages, as part of your pathology report, Ki-67 will automatically be included in that panel of testing.)

Cell Grade

Just as your teachers used to score your final exams at the end of every semester, your pathologist is going to score your cancer cells. The pathologist's scores are going to be based on the appearance as well as the growth patterns of the cells, and how these factors differ from those of healthy breast cells. While, like us, you always certainly wished for the highest score possible in school, in this case you are, in general, hoping for a low grade; note, however, like most everything to do with curing cancer, the grade of the cell alone does not determine a treatment path or an outcome: sometimes higher grade cancers are more easily treatable because certain treatments, such as chemotherapy and radiation, work by targeting rapidly dividing cells. In this case, higher-grade cancers are more vulnerable to treatment. 'Higher-grade' is a term that may correlate to 'poorly differentiated' and/or 'aggressive' when describing cancer cells. I have heard Julie say, in her irreverent fashion, that we doctors like to have at least three ways of saying the same thing, and we like to assign acronyms to each term. That way we sound really smart, and no one knows what we're talking about. This self-deprecating thinking is not without merit, but if you as the patient understand that the terms are quite similar, their subtle medical differences fade into the background as you participate in your treatment planning.

There are different grading systems for different types of cancer. For example, the Gleason system is used for prostate cancer, and the Fuhrman system for kidney cancer. For breast cancer, the Bloom-Richardson system is employed, and the possible scores are as follows:

- GX; a score of GX indicates that a grade cannot be assigned to the cancer cells in question.

- G1; Grade 1 (also called 'low grade' and 'well differentiated') cells look only slightly different from healthy cells, and they grow slowly (meaning few cells are dividing and making new cells), in organized patterns.

- G2; Grade 2 (also called 'intermediate grade,' 'moderate grade,' and 'modestly differentiated') cells are easily differentiated from healthy cells, and they are growing (dividing) somewhat faster than normal cells.

- G3; Grade 3 (also called 'high grade' and 'poorly differentiated') cells look substantially different from normal,

JULIE'S TIPS FOR TAKING CONTROL OF YOUR PATHOLOGY REPORT

1. Keep everything in one place.

The single most important gift you can give yourself during—and after—your cancer experience, is to reduce your stress level. Every day stress, of itself, is a cause of disease—and having her doctor say that she has cancer can jolt a girl's everyday stress levels right off the chart. So the idea is to create conditions in your life that control stress—to put yourself in a place where, when you need to put your hand on the results of one particular lab test or another, your hand will know right where to go.

Buy a special folder or binder to hold all of your cancer-related information. Mine was an inexpensive, three-ring pink binder my artistic ten-year-old daughter decorated with a flower motif, and inside were tabs for *Pathology Report, Chemo Schedule, Reconstruction Options, Insurance,* etc. Behind each tab were pages with pockets to hold documents such as the actual reports issued by the lab, and the copious paperwork that arrived in the mail from my insurer. I found the binder format especially efficient because I could keep my notes on three-ring paper, adding more pages as I needed to do that. You can go low-end as I did with my inexpensive, Target binder, high-end as one of my patients did who decided an ornate Italian leather notebook was exactly what she needed, and even high tech by keeping your notes on your laptop computer, or even on your iPhone with Apple's breast cancer diagnosis app.[1] It isn't the method of organization that's important, only the organization itself.

2. Make sure your information is portable.

Cancer treatment requires the expertise of a multidisciplinary cancer-fighting team. We'll talk more about the people who make up this team in Chapter Eight; for now, know that in the course of your recovery you'll be visiting general surgeons, oncologists, reconstruction surgeons, your breast cancer coordinator, and all of these different specialists will need a lot of the same information you've now organized in one place. Your binder or notebook or laptop is your easy reference resource, containing all the basic information on which your treatment is based; take it with you to each doctor's appointment. If you've decided to keep your information on your desktop computer: make sure you can easily transfer the info to a laptop or tablet so it can travel with you, too.

If you are seeking a second opinion about your diagnosis or care, you will need to take your binder or laptop with you to your appointment with the consulting physician.

3. Make sure to ask for copies of all your paper reports.

---

1 https://itunes.apple.com/us/app/breast-cancer-diagnosis-guide/id389683262?mt=8.

You have a legal right to all of your medical records—and it is easy enough for your doctor to provide you with a copy of all of your paper reports. Not all doctor's offices, however, have a policy of automatically supplying copies of test results to patients, so be sure to ask for them. You will want copies of:

- blood test results

- tissue test results

- imaging test reports

Some women also keep copies of the films or digital images from their mammograms or MRIs, though I am not convinced this is necessary or entirely efficient. Multiple images may be taken over the course of your treatment—so changes in the cancer can be monitored and compared—

and keeping track of versions can become confusing and cumbersome. For this reason, images are generally stored at the facility where they were taken and can be transferred if a patient decides to change facilities or seek a second opinion. If you would like to maintain copies of these images, however, I suggest you ask for them on CD rather than in a hard-copy format.

That said, *copies* of most film test results are acceptable, but the majority of doctors will want *original mammogram films* as these are the best images for them to use to evaluate the subtle indications of any cancer that is occurring. Some facilities are, shall we say, *reluctant* to release original film to the patient. Here is my advice in this situation: stand your ground. Be persistent. These are your mammogram films and you have every legal right to possess them and take them to whichever doctor or facility you choose.

4. Keep a summary.

Some of the information in your pathology report is so foundational—so critical to each specialist—I found it helpful to keep a summary. I just made a handwritten list of "the most asked questions" and taped it, with my answers, to the inside front cover of my binder:

- The stage of my cancer is:

- My cancer is invasive/non-invasive.

- My cancer is/is not metastasized.

- My lymph node status is:

- The size of my tumor is:

- The grade of my tumor is:

- My ER/PR/HER2 status is:

- My cancer is growing at the rate of:

5. Be patient.

As Tom Petty once said in a song lyric that is oh, so, sadly true: *The waiting is the hardest part.* I mean, having a breast cyst aspirated is no fun, even if the anticipation of the procedure is, indeed, in most cases, worse than the actual experience, but waiting days or a week to find out the result of the cell analysis from the aspirated fluid can be torturous. So get used to this upfront: while you will have the results of some tests back in your hands very quickly, most breast-cancer related tests take between three and seven days to arrive. The best practice is to simply ask when the result of each test your doctor orders will be available. Keeping track of the arrival dates of test results reduces your anxiety, prevents you from wondering if and why your doctor is not communicating with you, and is another great way to take control of your treatment.

But there is another reason to practice patience in relation to your breast cancer test results, and it is the temptation to fixate on the results of each one of the tests. The truth—the fine distinctions that comprise both the art and science of breast cancer treatment—is that to wholly understand each woman's unique manifestation of breast cancer and determine an appropriate treatment for it, she and her doctor need to be able to see the whole picture of the cancer. It is highly unlikely that the results of one test will tell you how to proceed with your cancer treatment; rather, the results of all your tests together will help you determine what road you will be traveling to your cure.

Finally, even if you should receive test results before your next appointment with your doctor, it is wise to wait to talk with her or him to interpret those results. For one thing, the medical language and shorthand used to compose a lab report is not always the most patient-friendly. While I am a huge advocate of using the Internet to gather information about pressing medical issues, I still advise that you wait until you have the opportunity to discuss your test results with your doctor before trying to come to a conclusion about what your test results are telling you. Your doctor is going to infuse the interpretation of your test results with knowledge and insight she has cultivated from experience with many different types of cancer and cancer treatments, as well as with first-hand knowledge of you and your unique cancer; the Internet can be a godsend in terms of providing a patient with solid background information, but it is not in anyone's imagination a substitute for an expert sitting in a chair beside you and discussing what is going on inside *you*.

There is a corollary to the patience rule here. Be willing to wait until your appointment to get answers to your questions. There is a process that a physician's mind goes through when they take in information, process it, and then make recommendations regarding treatment. Part of that process, a very important part of that process, involves being in the appropriate place, with the chart in front of us, and keyboard or pen in hand. When one of my patients sees me in the grocery store and asks a question about their medical care, I don't just change gears in order to answer. I cross four lanes of traffic and pull a screeching u-turn over a big concrete meridian in order to answer. I can do it, but it may not get my patient the very best answer, I may not consider all of the factors I would have liked to without the entire chart and my head in the "practice medicine" rather than "choose the correct lettuce" mode, and I probably won't remember to put the grocery store conversation in the chart the next time I get to the office. Again: be willing to wait until your appointment to get answers to your questions.

6. **Ask questions—ask as many questions and every question you need to ask.**

Let's say that your doctor does not order one or more of the tests that can be done for a conventional pathology report—you will likely want to know why, and *there is likely a very good reason.* Perhaps knowing the results of a particular test will not, at least for that particular moment in time, advance your understanding of the cancer you are dealing with? Be secure that, should your doctor eventually feel the need for additional testing, the tissue in question is kept at the lab for more tests later; mean-

time, ask for an explanation. Remember that you and your doctor are a cancer-fighting team, and any team works best when each member knows fully what all the other members know. When it comes to cancer, there really are very few silly questions, so ask, ask, ask away.

Another corollary to this rule is, there may be tests that you would like to have done that your doctor may not be thinking about doing. This is often especially true when you are using an integrative approach. MTHFR testing and vitamin D3 levels are just a couple of labs that are routinely available but might not be part of every doctor's cancer workup, but they can be critically important to the integrative approach. Ask, ask, ask.

healthy cells; a high percentage of the cells are dividing, meaning they grow rapidly, and in irregular and disorganized patterns.

- **G4**; Grade 4 (also called 'undifferentiated') cells are the highest graded cancer cells.

You want to be careful not to confuse the 'grade' of your cancer with its 'stage.' Grade is based on the appearance of the cells, and their patterns of growth. The stage of a cancer, which we'll talk about in the next few paragraphs, is based on the size of the cancer, and how far it has or has not spread beyond its site or origin.

Size of the Breast Cancer

This is an exceptionally clear-cut characteristic: just how big is the tumor we're talking about? Cancer is measured in millimeters (one millimeter equals .04 inch) or centimeters (one centimeter equals one quarter of an inch). Pull your ruler out of your drawer: a one-centimeter tumor is quite small, while a five-centimeter (two inch) tumor can seem (and feel) terribly alarming. The size of the tumor will help determine the stage of the cancer but, like so many other things in life: *size alone does not matter*. A large tumor can take up a lot of space but be, actually, the gentlest of giants—a lumbering and sloppy but harmless Golden Retriever; a small tumor can be a sweet, loveable little Shih Tzu that yaps its way into a frenzy of aggression.

Stages of Breast Cancer

The stage of a cancer is most commonly expressed as a number on a scale of zero through four, usually as a Roman numeral, and is determined, as we have already discussed, by its size as well as how far it has spread from its site of origin, specifically: Is the cancer invasive or non-invasive? Has it spread to the lymph nodes? Has it spread beyond the breast to other parts of the body? Often you'll hear your doctor and other health professionals talk about the distance a breast cancer has spread in terms of 'local' cancer (cancer that is confined within the breast), 'regional' cancer (cancer that has migrated to the lymph nodes, especially those in the armpit), and 'distant' or metastatic cancer (cancer that has migrated to other parts of the body, beyond the breast).

Why does your doctor stage your cancer? Staging helps both doctor and patient draw a baseline under the common experience of breast cancer and how that common experience differs or is similar to the experience of one particular patient. Employing a common language, and looking to common milestones, can help you and your cancer fighting team interpret the results contained in your pathology report, and make treatment decisions.

● **Stage 0 (Carcinoma in situ)** is used to describe non-invasive cancer in which there is no evidence of cancer cells, or other abnormal cells that are not themselves cancerous, moving away from the site at which they originated or infiltrating neighboring tissue. Examples include DCIS, LCIS, Paget's disease.

● **Stage I** is used to describe an invasive cancer, typically 'microscopic invasion', in which the cancer cells have just begun to infiltrate tissue outside of the lobule or duct that is the point of origin. There are two sub-stages to Stage I:

  • *Stage IA*, in which a tumor of up to 2 centimeters in size is present, but the cancer has not spread outside the breast (that is, no lymph nodes are involved);

  • *Stage IB*, in which no tumor is present, but smaller groups of cancer cells (larger than .2 millimeter but no larger than 2 millimeters) have been discovered in the lymph nodes, OR a tumor is present in the breast that is no larger than 2 centimeters, and there are smaller groups of cancer cells (larger than 0.2 millimeter but no larger than 2 millimeters) in the lymph nodes.

● **Stage II** is used to describe an invasive cancer and there are also two sub-stages:

  • *Stage IIA*, in which no tumor can be detected in the breast, but groups of cancer cells larger than 2 millimeters are seen in the lymph nodes in the armpit (axillary) or under the breast bone (internal mammary), OR

~ a tumor is present in the breast that measures not more than 2 centimeters, and groups of cancer cells larger than 2 millimeters are seen in the lymph nodes in the armpit (axillary) or under the breast bone (internal mammary), OR

~ a tumor is present in the breast that measures larger than 2 centimeters but not larger than 5 centimeters, and groups of cancer cells have not spread to the lymph nodes in the armpit (axillary).

- *Stage IIB*, in which a tumor is present that measures larger than 2 centimeters but not larger than 5 centimeters, and cancer cells have spread to between one and three lymph nodes in the armpit (axillary) or under the breast bone (internal mammary), OR a tumor is present measures larger than 5 centimeters, but cancer cells have not spread to the lymph nodes in the armpit (axillary).

● **Stage III** is used to describe an invasive cancer and there are three sub-stages:

- *Stage IIIA*, in which no tumor is present, but cancer cells have spread to 4 to 9 lymph nodes in the armpit (axillary) or under the breast bone (internal mammary), OR

~ a tumor is present, of any size, and cancer cells
have spread to 4 to 9 lymph nodes in the armpit
(axillary) or under the breast bone (internal mammary), OR

~ a tumor larger than 5 centimeters is present and
cancer cells have spread to 1 to 3 lymph nodes
in the armpit (axillary) or under the breast bone
(internal mammary).

- *Stage IIIB*, in which a tumor of any size is present and
cancer cells have spread to the chest wall and/or the
skin of the breast and caused swelling or an ulcer, OR
the cancer has been diagnosed as *inflammatory breast
cancer*.

- *Stage IIIC*, in which there may be either no cancer
in the breast, or a tumor of any size, but cancer cells
have spread to the skin of the breast or the chest wall
and have also been discovered in the lymph nodes
either above or below the collarbone OR

~ cancer cells have been discovered in at least 1 or up
to 10 lymph nodes in the armpit (axillary) AND
the lymph nodes in the vicinity of the breastbone, OR

~ cancer cells have been discovered in 10 or more
lymph nodes in the axillary.

● Stage IV refers to invasive cancer in which cancer cells
have been discovered outside the breast and lymph nodes
in the armpit (axillary), and in other organs of the body—

the lungs, skin, bones, brain, liver—and/or distant lymph nodes. Stage IV is also referred to as 'advanced' or 'metastatic' cancer.

While the numerical staging system we've just outlined is the principal way in which breast cancer is described, there is another system called TNM that is sometimes employed. Briefly, this system is based on three characteristics of the cancer: the size of the tumor (T stands for tumor), the extent of lymph node involvement (N stands for node), and whether and to what extent the cancer has metastasized (M stands for metastasis). This method of staging is used primarily in clinical trials; for patients who are participating or considering participation in a clinical trial as part of their breast cancer journey, we refer you to the National Cancer Institute's excellent and detailed guide to this complex staging system.[III]

Tumor Necrosis

Tumor necrosis means that dead breast cancer cells have been found within the sample of tissue your pathologist is using for testing purposes. It is a predictor of aggressive cancer.

[III] http://www.cancer.gov/cancertopics/pdq/treatment/breast/healthprofessional/page3.

Surgical Margins

During breast cancer surgery—mastectomy, lumpectomy, or surgical biopsy—your doctor strives to remove the breast cancer as well as a 'rim' of normal, healthy tissue around the cancerous tissue. This rim is called the 'surgical margin' or the 'margin of resection.' She does this in order to be as certain as possible that all of the cancer has been taken away. After surgery—sometimes *during* surgery—your pathologist will examine the rim to determine if there are cancer cells present in it; your pathology report will include his findings, which he will note in one of three ways:

- A notation of 'Clear,' 'Negative,' or 'Clean' means that no cancer cells were discovered at the outermost edge of the rim of healthy tissue; in some cases, the pathologist will supply an actual measurement of the distance between the outermost edge of the rim and the cancerous tissue. When 'Clear' is noted, additional surgery is rarely required.

- A notation of 'Positive' means that the cancer cells abut the outermost edge of the excised tissue; in this case your doctor will most likely recommend additional surgery to remove additional, remaining cancer cells.

- A notation of 'Close' means that your pathologist discovered cancer cells very close to the outermost edge of the healthy tissue, but not at the edge itself. In this case, you and your doctor can decide if you are comfortable with the margin or if more surgery is necessary.

What is critical to note in regard to surgical margins is that there is no standard margin to which all doctors routinely adhere. The standard changes from hospital to hospital, with some hospitals requiring a two-millimeter margin to achieve a 'clear' notation and others a one-millimeter margin for the same designation. Your doctor's comfort with the margin will determine her recommendation for additional surgery. In addition, it may impact the course of chemotherapy your oncologist will recommend; if, in your case, chemo is after surgery, it is important that you ask your doctor at an early stage in your treatment how 'clear' will be defined by your surgical team.

Vascular or Lymphatic System Invasion

As we discussed back in Chapter One, about breast anatomy, there are two systems that channel nutrients to your breasts and cellular waste products out of them: the vascular system, which moves blood through your body, and the lymphatic system, which moves lymphatic fluid. Sometimes breast cancer cells will break through the walls of the vessels that carry the blood and/or the lymphatic fluid, and this can increase the risk of the abnormal cells traveling to other parts of the body, or of the cancer recurring again after an initial successful treatment. If the cancer cells have invaded the vascular or the lymphatic system, your pathology report will indicate 'present' and, if there is no evidence of an invasion, your report will indicate 'absent.'

Note that 'lymphatic system invasion' and 'lymph node involvement' are two issues, separate and distinct.

Lymph Node Involvement

Strategically placed along the body's lymphatic channels are *lymph nodes*—small, oval-shaped organs whose job it is to filter the lymphatic fluid. The armpit, or axillary, lymph nodes and the internal mammary lymph nodes filter the lymph fluid as it leaves the breast; one of the functions of this filter system is to try to capture cancer cells before they can leave the breast and migrate to other parts of the body.

Sometimes before and sometimes during surgery for invasive breast cancer, the surgeon removes at least one, and frequently more, of the underarm lymph nodes. These nodes are then examined to discover if they contain cancer cells. When the nodes are clear, clean or free of cancer, your pathologist will indicate that your cancer is 'negative' regarding *lymph node involvement*. When there are cancer cells in the nodes, your pathologist will return a 'positive' result; this can mean that the cancer has been trying to spread out of the breast, and suggest an increased risk that it has.

In addition to noting whether the general test result is positive or negative, your report will indicate the number of nodes that were removed and, of those, the number that tested positive for cancer cells. To interpret this result, look at the two numbers on the report that are separated by a slash mark. The first number refers to the number of nodes that contained cancer and the second to the total number of nodes that were removed for testing. That is, if two nodes were removed, and none of them tested positive for cancer cells, your result would be 0/2. If five nodes were removed and two of them tested positive for cancer cells, your result would be 2/5.

In addition to telling you the number of nodes that tested positive, your pathologist will also indicate how much cancer is contained in the nodes. You may find this value expressed in your report as the letter 'N' (for 'node') followed by a numeral:

- N1, meaning that cancer has been found in one to three lymph nodes in the underarm area;

- N2, meaning that cancer has been found in four to nine nodes in the underarm area;

- N3, meaning that cancer has been found in ten or more nodes in the underarm area, or that the cancer has spread under or over the collarbone area.

She may also, or alternatively, express the value by indicating that the cancer cells found in the lymph nodes are:

- 'microscopic,' meaning only a few cancer cells were found in the nodes and the risk that the cancer has spread is 'minimal,' and a microscope is needed to detect the cancer;

- 'macroscopic,' 'gross,' or 'significant,' meaning there is a substantial amount of cancer in the node or nodes, and the presence of cancer can be felt, or detected without a microscope;

- 'extracapsular extension,' meaning the cancer has spread or begun to spread outside the wall of the node.

Ploidy

The unusual word 'ploidy' refers to the number of sets of chromosomes in the nucleus of a cell. Recall that chromosomes are the structures within a cell that contain the material that is our genetic blueprint—our DNA—and that a normal, healthy cell carries two sets of twenty-three each or, in other words, a full set of chromosomes that includes a single copy of each gene. As cells grow, and divide, to create new cells, the chromosomes have a critical role to play in assuring that the DNA of the cell is copied correctly into both of the new cells. As we discussed in Chapter Four, cancer begins when the DNA is copied incorrectly so, as part of your diagnosis, your doctor may want to know if your cancer cells contain the correct amount of DNA. We say *may* because this test is not routinely performed and may not be a part of your pathology report; this is because medical experts don't yet agree on how to use the results of this test to determine treatment options. If your doctor does believe ploidy can help to provide you with information that will empower treatment decisions, she will order a test in which your pathologist will look at your cancer cells under a microscope and report one of two results:

● **Diploid,** which means that the greater proportion of your cancer cells have the same number of chromosomes as healthy cells. This can indicate a slower-growing, or less aggressive, cancer.

● **Aneuploid,** which means that the greater proportion of your cancer cells have an incorrect number of chromosomes—too many, or too few. This many indicate that the cancer is faster-growing, or more aggressive.

Hormone Receptor Status

Determining your hormone receptor status is a major part of charting your breast cancer treatment course. This is because the growth of some breast cancers is influenced by hormones—either *estrogen* or *progesterone*, two hormones that occur naturally in the female human body. Your pathologist will perform a *hormone receptor assay*, which is a test that tells you whether or not your breast cancer cells contain specific proteins that act as receptors for these hormones—that is, do they contain the specific protein that picks up signals from either estrogen or progesterone that tells the cells to grow.

This test is critical because it can be fundamental in deciding the type of treatment you opt for. Approximately two out of three breast cancer patients will test positive for hormone receptors and, if you are one of that majority, you and your doctor can discuss including hormonal therapy as part of your treatment plan. We'll discuss hormone therapy for breast cancer in more detail in Chapter Eleven; for now note that this therapy can include medications that lower the amount of estrogen in your body or, alternatively, block the estrogen in the body from attaching to its receptors on cell surfaces and supporting the growth of the cancer cells. These sorts of medications can slow or even stop the growth of hormone receptive cancers.

- A result of *estrogen-receptor-positive* (ER+) means that the cancer has receptors for estrogen, and suggests that the cells receive signals from the hormone estrogen that promotes their growth.

- A result of *progesterone-receptor-positive* (PR+) means that the cancer has receptors for progesterone, and suggests that the cells receive signals from the hormone progesterone that promotes their growth.

- A result of *hormone-receptor-negative* means that no receptors are present in the cancer cells; any sort of hormone therapy will likely be ineffective in this case and you and your doctor will want to focus on choosing other treatment options.

Additionally, there is some evidence that hormone receptor status is related to the risk of cancer recurrence after treatment: tumors that are hormone positive recur slightly less frequently than do tumors that are hormone negative,[112] although after a period of five years the difference in risk begins to decrease.

HER2 Status

The hormone receptors we talked about in the previous section are, of course, not the only proteins that may or may not be

---

112 http://www.ncbi.nlm.nih.gov/pubmed/17960621.

present (or may or may not be present in correct quantities) in a cell—the body is a complex creation and, while its biochemical logic is always elegant, it is rarely simple. Our genetic code contains all sorts of prompts for our cells to create any number of proteins they need to function in a normal, healthy way.

HER2, or *Human Epidermal Growth Factor Receptor 2*, is one of the genes that may contribute to the development of breast cancer, and your pathology report will almost always contain information about whether or not this is true in your case.

Let's follow the path of HER2: HER2 is a gene that prompts our cells to produce HER2 protein. What do the HER2 proteins do? They are members of a family of growth factors that regulate how normal breast cells grow, divide, and repair themselves. Do you remember Dennis the Menace? His mother might be making cookies at her house, and Mrs. Wilson might be making cookies in hers. Dennis could walk into either kitchen, or both, asking to help, and instead of helping his family to get the job done, both kitchens were a disaster. There was flour in his mom's hair and on Mrs. Wilson's face, cookies were burning, the fire department was pulling up outside the house, and all sense of propriety and order had evaporated. HER2 can be a Dennis the Menace-like influence on the Epidermal Growth Factor Family. In approximately one quarter of all breast cancer cases, however, the HER2 gene isn't functioning properly: it is making too many copies of itself, which is known as HER2 gene amplification (the proverbial "help" from Dennis the Menace). This overproduction of the genetic copies causes, in turn, the breast cells to make far too many receptor proteins—as many receptors as the cells think they need to make to receive all of that overflow of the HER2 gene. This is known as HER2 protein overexpression, and the result of it is that normal breast cells begin to grow and divide uncontrollably.

If your pathology report indicates that your cancer is HER2-positive, it means that your pathologist has found evidence that HER2 gene amplification or HER2 protein overexpression is occurring. Cancers that are designated HER2-positive tend to grow faster and are more likely to both spread and recur, when compared to cancers that are HER2-negative.

There are special medications designed specifically to treat HER2-positive cancers, and we will discuss those in more depth in Chapter Thirteen; for now, let's stick to the narrower scope of this chapter—how to interpret your pathology report—because there are several caveats you'll want to keep in mind about HER2 testing.

The first is that there are four different tests that might be used to test your cancer for HER2, and how the results will appear on your particular pathology report will depend on the test your pathologist has employed:

● **The ImmunoHistoChemistry test (IHC test)** discovers if there is too much HER2 protein in the cancer cells. The results you receive will be noted as 0, meaning no protein was discovered; 1+, which is also a negative result; 2+,

which means that the cells are on the borderline of producing too much protein; 3+, which is a positive result
meaning that the pathologist has discovered HER2 protein overexpression.

- **The Fluorescence In Situ Hybridization,** or FISH test,
discovers if there are too many copies of the HER2 gene
within the cancer cells. If this is the test your pathologist
uses you will receive results indicating the test had a positive outcome (meaning there is HER2 gene amplification in the cells), or negative outcome (meaning there is
no HER2 gene amplification in the cells). Sometimes a
FISH test is ordered for those patients who have an IHC
result of 2+ since they are on the borderline, so an actual
positive or negative distinction can be made.

- **The Subtraction Probe Technology Chromogenic In
Situ Hybridization,** or SPoT-Light HER2 CISH test,
like the FISH test, discovers if there are too many copies
of the HER2 gene in the cancer cells. Again, as with the
FISH test, the results will be either a positive notation,
meaning there is HER2 gene amplification present, or a
negative notation, meaning there is not.

- **The Inform Dual In Situ Hybridization test,** or the
Inform HER2 Dual ISH test, works in the same way as
the two tests previously noted, by discovering if there are
too many copies of the HER2 gene in the cancer cells;

once again the results will be either positive (indicating HER2 gene amplification) or negative (indicating no HER2 gene).

Of these four tests, why will a doctor order one over the other? Well, unfortunately, which test is run is not always within your doctor's control: often the sort of test you receive will depend upon which laboratory your pathologist is affiliated with, his or her preferences and the laboratory's standards and/or capabilities. One laboratory may have different criteria or rules for classifying HER2 test results; one pathologist may employ a different standard in deciding whether to apply a positive or a negative status. Often these more subjective applications of standards come into play when the test results are not clear-cut—somewhere in between negative and positive, the gray area where medicine becomes less of a science and more of an art; other times, discrepancies in determining an HER2 test result can be *strictly* science, as tissue from one area of a breast can test HER2-negative while tissue from a different area of the very same breast can test positive.

That said, it is to your benefit to know which sort of HER2 test you have had for a variety of reasons. For example, medicines that target HER2-positive breast cancers will generally be prescribed only for the following results: IHC 3+, FISH positive, SPoT-Light HER2 CISH positive, and Inform HER2 Dual ISH positive—and this is because the cancers that provoke these results have proven to respond best to these medications. Unfortunately, not all of these four tests are equally accurate. The IHC test is less reliable than the other three; if, for example, you have received the IHC test and your result is 2+ (that is, your cells are on the 'borderline' of producing too much HER2 protein), you will want to ask your doctor to have one of the other three, more precise tests performed to determine if you are a candidate for specialized HER2-positive treatment.

A further HER2 complication is that cancers that, at one time, test HER2-positive can become HER2-negative, and, just the opposite, cancers that at one time presented as HER2-negative can become HER2-positive. If your breast cancer has recurred, you and your doctor will likely want to order a new biopsy in order to run a new HER2 status test rather than relying on the results of the initial test to influence current treatment decisions.

Triple-Negative Breast Cancer

Somewhere between 10 and 20% of breast cancer patients will receive the diagnosis that their cancer is 'triple negative.' This means that their pathology reports will indicate they have tested negative for estrogen receptors (they are *ER-*), progesterone receptors (they are *PR-*), and HER2 (they are *HER2-*). Their cancers, in other words, are not promoted by either of the hormones estrogen or progesterone, nor by too much HER2 proteins—and this means that hormonal cancer therapies, and therapies that target HER2 receptors, are likely to be ineffective in treating this particular cancer and special 'triple negative medicines' are a better choice for treatment.

EGFR Status

EGFR stands for *Epidermal Growth Factor Receptor*, a gene that is sometimes called the HER1 gene. As with the HER2 gene, EGFR and the protein it makes may influence how a particular manifestation of breast cancer progresses, and the sorts of treatment that might be most appropriate for it. We use the words 'may' and 'might' in this context cautiously, however. While it is indeed possible for your pathologist to determine if there are too many copies of the EGFR gene present in a sample of breast cancer cells—and therefore EGFR amplification in progress—EGFR-targeted treatment for breast cancer is far from settled. If your doctor has ordered an EGFR test as part of your lab work, your pathology report will indicate that your cancer is 'EGFR-positive,' 'EGFR-negative,' or, possibly, 'undetermined,' meaning your pathologist cannot make a clear determination based on the sample tissue with which he was working. But what will these designations mean in terms of how you will act upon them? While some cancers, such as colon cancer and lung cancer, respond to medications that target EGFR issues, breast cancer response to EGFR-targeted treatment is still a matter under study. Needless to say, a patient's EGFR status is not routinely a part of standard pathology reporting.

BRCA1 and BRCA 2 Testing, and Beyond…

As EGFR is not, as of the 2013 edition of this book, a routine part of pathology reporting, neither is BRCA1 and BRCA2 testing. We include it here because testing for the abnormal BRCA genes is certainly on its way to becoming routine, at least for a select portion of breast cancer and *potential* breast cancer patients. For the purposes of this chapter we are limiting ourselves to discussion of the tests themselves and not to the implications of the availability of such predictive tests.

As we have already discussed, heredity can be a 'risk factor' in terms of developing disease—from heart disease to Alzheimer's to diabetes to breast cancer. While it is true that the majority of people who do develop breast cancer have no family history of it, scientists have been able to pin down the roots of most of the cases of breast cancer that *are* inherited. These roots are the BRCA1 (BReast CAncer gene 1) and BRCA2 (BReast CAncer gene 2); both belong to a class of genes known as tumor suppressors. Women and men who inherit a mutation of either of these genes—a mutation that can be inherited both maternally and paternally—have a much greater than average lifetime risk of developing breast cancer as well as, in the case of women, ovarian cancer. Here's the tricky part, however: just because a person might test positive for the gene does not mean that he or she will automatically develop the disease.

We recommend further reading, including the National Cancer Institute's guide to genetic testing,[113] if you are considering requesting this test. If you decide to do so, or if your doctor recommends that you do, based on her knowledge of your family history, note that the test cannot be conducted on tissue samples that will likely have already been gathered via biopsy. Rather, the patient must undergo a special blood test.

In the same category are other genetic tests that have taken disease diagnosis and treatment to a level once reserved for futuristic fiction. These tests are known as genomic assays. A genomic assay is a test that uses a tissue sample to analyze the activity of a whole group of genes, versus the activity of one gene within any group. Knowing which genes are present in the tissue (or not present) and being able to estimate their population and activity level can help you and your doctor hone in on the most efficacious treatment options, and can also help your doctor predict, and plan for, recurrence. For example, a patient might choose to undergo chemotherapy even as it is less necessary for recovery from a current diagnosis, if the treatment can reduce a high recurrence risk factor.

There are currently three tests that a doctor can order for breast cancer patients:

---

113 http://www.cancer.gov/cancertopics/factsheet/Risk/BRCA.

- **The Oncotype DX test,** which analyzes the activity of twenty-one different genes and is an option for women with early-stage, hormone-receptor-positive breast cancer.

- **The MammaPrint test,** which analyzes seventy different genes and is an option for women who are diagnosed with early-stage breast cancer, either hormone-receptor-positive or hormone-receptor-negative.

- **The Mammostrat test,** which measures the activity levels of five genes and is recommended for women with early-stage, hormone-receptor-positive breast cancer.

Keep in mind: if you and your doctor choose to take advantage of cutting-edge genetic testing to inform treatment and/or risk assessment, even such advanced and sophisticated tests cannot be interpreted in isolation. None of the tests in your pathology report can or should, standing alone, determine your course of treatment. Moreover, accurately interpreting test results—and coming to appropriate, efficacious, and satisfying treatment decisions—requires discussion between, at the very least, two very important people: you and your doctor.

8

Let's Get Real

Things I Wish Someone Had Told Me When I Got Cancer

You, yourself, as much as anybody in the entire universe, deserve your love and affection.

Buddha

This is a truth I didn't learn until I got sick: even when you don't have cancer, you've got to pour love on yourself.

Julie

I have already talked about my can-cer as a gift—I mean, let's face it, at this point I was going to have cancer whether I liked it or not, so why not embrace it as an opportunity to change my life, for the better, all at once? I'm not saying I didn't feel it was my right to indulge in the alternatives—sorrow, anger, and even self-pity—at least for a moment here and there, especially when I was first diagnosed, but sorrow, anger and self-pity do not constitute a long-term plan. My long-term plan was to beat the crap out of cancer, and get on with living the life I love.

In order to fight the good fight, however, I knew I needed to be prepared for what was ahead. I needed a game plan. A to-do list. And I wanted each item on my to-do list to be part of an overarching agenda, or attitude, that focused not on the negative, not on the disease I was dealing with, but on the positive lifestyle changes I could now, without guilt, allow myself.

Like most women with a busy schedule—and, let's face it, that is most women—I had always put myself and my needs last. The kids needed help with homework? My husband had a hard day at the office? My mom needed to get to a dentist appointment? Someone on my staff needed a day off? No problem! I was there to offer tutoring in seventh grade math, be a sounding board, give a ride, fill in. But what happens when your needs come after everyone else's is that, often, 'after' never comes. There are only so many hours in a day, after all. Sometimes it's just easier to flop into bed at the end of the day and promise yourself that *tomorrow* you'll make time for a massage, an hour of reading, a glass of wine with your girlfriends.

This I-come-last way of thinking leads to a risky set of behaviors. When we come last we don't eat right, we don't get enough exercise, our stress levels sky rocket because we make solving other people's problems more important than solving our own, and a lot of us even give up sleep to do it. Many of us rationalize these risky behaviors with the thought that we are making sacrifices out of love for our families and our wish to care for them as completely as we can. In our haste and determination to serve, however, the irony can go over our heads: risky behaviors make us sick and deplete our ability to do the very things that are most important to us.

So here was the message I needed to hear, the meditation I needed to repeat to myself every day until it was so much a part of me it was second nature: *I come first*. I have to admit, even now, after practicing this for many, many months, it's hard to write that down because it sounds so selfish. But it's not selfish at all. It's self-preservation. In my first book, *Healing Our Autistic Children*, I likened this I-come-first approach to life to advice that every one of us hears every time we get on a plane: if the cabin pressure drops, and that crazy yellow airbag falls from the ceiling, and you've got a child with you, put your own mask on before you try to help your child put on hers. Why? Because if you can't breathe you will panic or pass out, and then you will be of no use to anyone else who needs help, including your own child. I've got a big smile on my face as I tell you now that—thank you very much for the hard lesson, cancer—I have at last fully internalized my own advice.

I come first is a huge shift for most of us to make, but, as I said, it isn't a selfish one at all; simply put, I had to make the conscious choice to start treating myself at least as well as I treated everyone else. I am asking you to make that same choice now. Decide to really just love yourself; all your other choices, and the hard work it will take to implement them, will follow from this simple, overarching attitude: I love *me*.

I think it is important—perhaps even critical—to point out that part of living the I-come-first lifestyle is feeling empowered to make the choices that *you* truly want to make. I am offering a great deal of advice in this book. All of the advice flows from my personal experience of cancer, the medical residency I put myself through upon my diagnosis, and the combined medical expertise of myself and my co-author Ankit and the science that backs up the expertise. All of that said, however, you are the only one who is walking in your shoes, and some of the decisions I made or that another doctor recommends are not going to be right for you. I pushed back against traditional treatment options by insisting that my mastectomies be done at the same time as my breast reconstruction surgery—a practice that was unusual just a few years ago but which is now becoming ever more common. This was the right decision for me, but it may not be for you. And there are legitimate reasons for why it may not be right—but only you will be able to decide if those reasons are legitimate *for you*, as you create your personal healing plan. Don't be afraid to ask questions and, when you have gathered the information you need, don't be afraid to make the decision that is healthiest and most comfortable for you.

As a cancer patient, what are the overarching ways in which you can show yourself affection? To prepare to heal and then to stay well? I think there are three steps.

1. Know about and understand what it will take to beat cancer, and make peace with the changes that you will be going through.

2. Put together a Super Bowl-caliber healing team.

3. Set positive, post-cancer goals.

Know and understand what it will take to beat cancer.

Every woman's experience with breast cancer will be different. Where the cancer is located within the breast and at what stage the cancer is when you are diagnosed are two of the biggest factors that will determine what your unique treatment plan will be. But how old you are when you are diagnosed, if you are married and/or if you have children, whether or not you have a flexible job schedule—these are also important factors and will weigh on the decisions that are ahead.

For most of us patients, the decisions we will have to make will revolve around three traditional treatment options: surgery, radiation, and/or chemotherapy. As a doctor, I thought I had an advantage going into treatment—I thought I'd have a naturally deeper understanding of how to prepare myself for coping with these options. As it turned out, my experience as a patient has made me a better doctor: even with my medical background, I found out I did not plan as well as I could have. Another gift cancer has given me is the opportunity to pass along what I have learned.

Chemotherapy

Chemo is a common part of cancer treatment, of course. It works by introducing chemicals into the body that kill the cancer cells. It can be used as a primary therapy, with the goal of curing the cancer, or in conjunction with surgery, to kill any cancers that might remain in the body after surgery and, used in this way, it is called *adjuvant* therapy. It can also be used to shrink a tumor in preparation for other treatments, such as surgery or radiation, to increase the efficacy of those treatments, in which case it is referred to as *neoadjuvant* therapy. Finally, chemotherapy can also be used in cases of advanced cancer to help relieve and control pain and, in such cases, is called *palliative* chemotherapy.

Chemotherapy and Your Sense of Smell

For me, chemo was the hardest part of my treatment and it was hard, in great part, because I had never been in a chemo room before I entered one as a patient. I was not prepared for what I found there. Chemo rooms are miserable places, and that is primarily because they stink. They stink of the *chemicals* that make up the *chemo* drugs that are being used in the room. They stink of the fragrances that are added to the cleaning products that are used in the room—in my case, baby powder; before chemo the aroma of baby powder would trigger pleasant memories of when my children were just born; after chemo, and I mean for a good three years after chemo, the odor of baby powder triggered nausea. They stink of the plastic containers in which the fluids are sterilized and, once the solution is circulating in your body, you can smell *and taste* the plastic in which the saline has been packaged.

The sense of smell is visceral, and primitive, one of the most acute memory triggers we humans have. It is also one of the senses most affected by chemo. The odor of the chemo room stayed with me long after my treatment: I couldn't drink bottled water for three years because it smelled funny—like plastic.

If you were a fan of the TV show *Sex and the City*, you'll remember that when Samantha was diagnosed with breast cancer, there was a scene of all the girls gathered in her chemo room, smiling and laughing and toasting with popsicles instead of the group's standard Cosmos. That's a nice image of supportive friends but, trust me, no one is ever that carefree in a chemo room, and I wish someone had been upfront with me about the impending assault on my senses before I began my treatment. That is why I am being so direct here. I wish I'd had some advance warning of how disgusting the smells, and tastes, of that room were going to be—because you can prepare for only those things you can expect. I wish someone had told me what a kick in the gut it was going to be to walk into a huge room, sit down in a recliner and see people of all ages and all stages of all cancers experiencing varying amounts of bald and pale and nausea and weight loss and death—and life. Even better, I wish I'd had some sort of a tool to get over the aversion—some training so that I could have learned to replace the smells, and tastes and sights and sounds with happier ones. I quickly learned to focus very internally on healing and sleeping while I was there. Hypnotherapy and self-hypnosis, which are relaxation methods that use deeply focused concentration to evoke calm and alter negative behaviors, can be powerful tools in combatting not only the anxiety and nausea that can be associated with undergoing chemotherapy;[114] I believe they can be employed to combat the negative and lingering assaults chemo imposes on our senses. How would this work? A friend

---

114 *http://www.cancer.org/treatment/treatmentsandsideeffects/
complementaryandalternativemedicine/mindbodyandspirit/hypnosis.*

recently quit smoking—hip, hip, hurrah!—and she used self-hypnosis in the process. She trained herself to be repulsed rather than attracted to the smell of cigarette smoke by focusing on the cleanliness and healthiness of the atmosphere in her home in the absence of the smoke residue. In the same way, by focusing on the benefits of chemo to the healing process, it may be possible to replace the negative associations of its smells and tastes with more positive ones.

If I had the opportunity to prepare again, I think I would use the technique I was taught the year after my father died. I was nineteen when he died of very aggressive leukemia. In the months after he transitioned from here to what I believe comes next, every time I thought of him, and I thought of him a lot, I was haunted by what his body looked like the day he died—he was no longer my vibrant brilliant bossy demanding loving Daddy, but a man whose body had wasted away to a mere replica of himself, still tall but very skinny and pale-as-the-sheets-of-the-hospital-bed. A year later, I learned some fabulous coping techniques that I didn't know I'd need later in my life to deal with my own chemo. I learned how to deliberately and consciously reject the memory of my dad's body in that bed, and instead to replace it with a visualization of one of the happiest times I could remember with him—a snapshot of joy and peace.

I wish I had remembered that technique, because here's how I would have employed it: I would have assessed the sight, the sound, the smell, the taste, and the touch of the experience in the chemo room. I would have looked at myself as I lost my hair and grew pale, would have looked at the other people in that room, and would have closed my eyes, replacing those images with a visualization of each of us whole and healthy and happy, probably walking the beach. I would have tuned the crushing silence, solicitous nurses and whispered voices of patients into a different symphony of music I love and can play in my head. I would have thought about each individual odor and taste and found something positive and happy to associate it with. And no matter how challenging it was, I would have visually asserted the happy thought whenever I experienced those smells or tastes.

Bathing During Chemo

I also discovered that I had not planned well enough for the simple act of bathing during chemo. Chemo can cause skin problems such as itching, rashes, allergic reactions, and sensitivity to sunlight, and there are specific ways to alleviate the problems. If, like me, you enjoy long, hot baths or showers, you should know going into chemo that, while long, hot baths and showers can be pleasurable, they can also dry out your skin. So, during chemo, you should opt for shorter, lukewarm showers and baths. To prevent or relieve itching or rashes, you will want to make sure you use a mild soap—one that is hypoallergenic, fragrance-free, glycerin-based, and/or contains colloidal oatmeal which can help soothe. You may also find that cornstarch can help with itching, but don't use baby powder as most brands contain ingredients that can be irritating to sensitive skin. Moisturizing with a fragrance-free, organic lotion after bathing will also help with sensitive skin issues, and using a lotion with SPF protection of at least 15 if you plan to be outdoors will help with sun sensitivity. Having learned from experience, I'd be sure to buy small containers of everything while I was figuring out what products worked for me; even some of the fragrance-free products had odors or textures that I didn't always like and, of course, adding insult to injury, what I could tolerate through the first chemo was revolting with the second one, and so on.

Here is one last tip for grooming during chemo: shave your legs before every chemo session. When your white cell counts fall after a chemo treatment (a side effect we will discuss in a few pages), you won't be able to use a razor. Even when the hair on my head fell out the hair on my legs continued to grow rather lushly for quite a while, and I was caught for most of a hot Florida summer having to choose between hairy legs and trying to shave with an electric razor—not a happy selection to have to make!

One thing I didn't have to worry about when bathing was my *port*.

Your Chemotherapy Port

When chemotherapy is a part of your cancer treatment, a portacath, or a port, a small device that is installed beneath the skin, usually just below the collarbone, is often surgically placed. The port has a catheter that connects it to a vein, and a small septum, or separate compartment, through which medicine can be inserted into the body and blood can be drawn out. Trust me on this: your port is going to make your life so much easier. Chemotherapy drugs are given intravenously, but chemotherapy is hard on the veins, and can scar them, and it often causes dehydration, so getting repeated IVs in your peripheral arm and hand veins can become difficult. You will become what is known to those of us in the medical profession as "a tough stick," meaning the nurse can't find a viable vein to plug the needle into. With a port, your oncologist never has to worry about accessing a vein for treatment; and, for this reason, you will actually come to love your port.

You may wonder what the difference is between a port and a PICC line. A PICC line—or peripherally inserted central catheter—is a slender, flexible tube that is inserted into a peripheral vein, usually on the underside of the upper arm, that allows your medical team intravenous access by terminating into a large vein near the heart. But, unlike a port that is inserted under the skin, a PICC line sits on the surface of the skin. That is, while the port is essentially a pierceable well beneath the skin, the PICC line is external. One has to be very careful about maintaining a PICC line, particularly when bathing, to make sure it doesn't get wet. With a port, on the other hand, there is no home maintenance, except possibly keeping it covered with a Band-Aid when it has recently been accessed.

You will likely keep your port for a period of four to six months, or about as long as your course of chemotherapy lasts. You may grow to like the convenience of your port and want to keep it longer—it is not unheard of for patients to keep their port for several years if they are continuing to use them regularly—but the downside of a port is that it can become infected. The other potential hazard that can arise when the port gets old is that there is always the possibility of mechanical failure. As much as they may joke about it, surgeons and radiologists are not happy about having to "fish" floating port parts out of their patients, no matter how rarely it may occur. Because the catheter's central line runs so close to the heart, the consequences of these issues can be dangerous, so your doctor will be very picky about how and who touches your port, and want to remove it as early as is convenient, given your treatment plan.

Chemotherapy and Your Blood Counts

During chemo your doctor will closely monitor your blood counts. This is because chemo not only kills cancer cells, it kills blood cells, too.

For example, white blood cells. There are five different types of white blood cells: neutrophils, eosinophils, basophils, lymphocytes, and monocytes. While these white blood cells all have qualities in common, they each have distinct functions. The white blood cell your doctor will worry most about when chemotherapy causes your total white count to drop are the neutrophils, also called the PMN cells. When you don't have enough of them, a condition known as neutropenia (lack of neutrophils) results. Neutrophils are critically important as the first line of defense for your body when fighting off a bacterial infection. This is why, for a good week to ten days after each chemo treatment, your doctor will instruct you to be extremely careful about any source of bacteria. You will be advised not to travel, not to eat raw food, not to be around sick people, not to have sex, not to shave your legs, and not to accept the lovely fresh flowers your friends may think to send to you to cheer you up.[115]

During chemo your platelets—the components of your blood that helps to stop bleeding—can drop as well, sometimes to the point that your doctor will postpone your chemo treatment until their level has risen. Similarly, your hemoglobin level—the number of cells available to transport blood to the tissues and organs of your body—will drop, and your doctor might postpone chemo in this circumstance as well.

About a week, sometimes sooner, after each chemo treatment you will return to your doctor's office to get a shot that will help to rescue and restore your white blood cells. This shot hurts to get, and it makes your bones ache after you've received it. This is because white blood cells are made in the marrow, or centers, of the bone, and the shot mobilizes the marrow to manufacture the blood cells that you've lost through chemo.

---

115 When friends sent fresh flowers to me during this time, my daughter Dani took it upon herself to make drawings of the bouquets before we sent them on to cheer up the nurses at the nurses' station. It was a wonderful way for Dani to feel that she was participating in my healing process—and it was wonderful for me because I still have the drawings she made and, so, I still have the flowers my friends sent over three years ago. I can look at those three-year-old fresh flowers whenever I want to, and they still cheer me up!

Your hips, your legs, your arms will truly ache—sometimes I thought I could feel my marrow actually moving—but the thing that saved me after each of these shots was my hyperbaric chamber. I experienced much less pain after these restorative shots when I followed them up with a dive in the chamber, and I have heard that same report from every other cancer patient I've ever talked with who has used hyperbarics to help heal during her or his treatment.

Chemotherapy and Your Bowels

It's a damned if you do, damned if you don't sort of situation: chemotherapy causes diarrhea and nausea; the drugs that are given to combat nausea cause constipation. This does not mean, however, that you need to spend all your time either in the bathroom or hoping to the heavens you will need the bathroom soon. What can save you? Probiotics, probiotics, and more probiotics.

We all know that bacteria can cause illness, but not all bacteria are created equal; some bacteria are good for us. Probiotics is another name for the estimated 100 trillion individual live, beneficial microorganisms that live in every normal, healthy bowel. When the probiotics in your system are out of balance—that is when the bad bacteria out number the good bacteria—the bowel can become irritated, resulting in belly-aches and cramps, bloating and gas, diarrhea or constipation among other even more serious illnesses.

Moreover, when the bowel is compromised, the immune system is also compromised. This is because sixty to seventy percent of the human immune system is located within the digestive system! In fact, it is said that your immune system makes more decisions within your bowel in twenty-four hours than it makes within the rest of your body in an entire lifetime. An expansive network of lymphatic tissue know as GALT, or gut associated lymphatic tissue, lies within the gut wall, just one cell layer away from those trillions of probiotic bacteria. That immune system tissue is constantly making decisions about how to respond to the bacteria in our bowel, deciding if the bacteria are the good strangers, or if they are bad guys that are trying to cause an infection or to which we need to have an allergic reaction. The bottom line is that your immune system's competence is determined largely through the practice of continuously assessing the microbes living in your intestines.

If you are already using probiotics at the time you are diagnosed, great! If you aren't, start them the day you find your lump. Some sources of probiotics are:

● **Yogurt, kefir, and some soft cheeses,** though if you are lactose intolerant or adhere, as I do, to a casein-free diet, these won't be optimal options for you;

● **Sourdough bread,** though bread, of course, contains gluten;

- **Miso,** a fermented soy bean paste used as a flavoring, and tempeh, fermented soybean patties that are high in protein and can be substituted for meat, though soy contains natural estrogens;

- **Fermented vegetables,** such as sauerkraut and sour pickles;

- Good quality probiotic dietary supplements.

Additionally, *prebiotics* are foods that support or "feed" the good bacteria that are already living in your digestive tract. Consider eating foods that are rich in prebiotic properties such as legumes, asparagus, and bananas.

Nausea

This is a subject we've touched on in other portions of this book but, as it can be a prominent component of the cancer experience, it deserves a section all its own. Nausea, of course, is the sensation that you are going to be sick—mild cases can make you unable to eat, but more severe cases can cause actual vomiting. During the cancer experience there are any number of culprits that can cause the sensation. Chemotherapy can cause nausea. Radiation can cause nausea. Targeted treatments such as Herceptin and Tykerb can cause nausea, and certain hormonal therapies such as Aromasin, Femara, and Tamoxifen can cause nausea. Nausea can be caused by certain medications your doctor might prescribe to relieve pain caused by various cancer treatments—medications from Demerol to Aleve—and it can also be caused by *other* side effects of cancer treatments, including constipation. Knowing that you are likely going to have to deal with nausea at some point in your cancer journey, managing it becomes key.

Traditionally, nausea is managed by prescription. Zofran, a drug that works by blocking serotonin, and Phenergan, a drug that works by blocking histamine, are two common ones. As with all drugs, however, these remedies themselves come with a long list of side effects including constipation, headaches, severe dizziness and chest pain for the former, and seizures, blurred vision, and hallucinations for the latter.

If your nausea is severe, by all means talk to your doctor about a prescriptive solution, but know that there are other ways to manage nausea that don't come with such scary side effects.

- **Eat sitting up.** Humans are designed to eat while we are upright—eating while lying down can disrupt the digestive process.

- **Brush your teeth after eating.** This will prevent lingering tastes that may induce nausea.

- **Eat slowly,** so you don't get full before you *feel* full—it can take up to twenty minutes for your stomach to communicate with your brain that it's had enough to eat.

- **Eat small quantities** of dry foods like toast or crackers several times a day to settle your stomach, and stay away from fried or other greasy foods as too much fat can trigger nausea.

- **Consider ordering in** rather than cooking at home. Sometimes just the smells of food, such as those that linger after cooking, can trigger nausea, so be thankful when friends, neighbors, and members of your church family bring already-cooked meals to your home.

- **Snack on ginger!** Ginger is both delicious and a classic remedy for nausea—I was a sailor before I was a doctor and I know of very few captains who will take a boat out on the water without a stock of ginger snaps in the galley. Munching ginger snaps or pickled ginger, sucking on candied ginger, sipping ginger tea, or even drinking ginger ale can be oh, so helpful.

- **Try taking magnesium supplements,** which have also been known to help with nausea.

- **Bear in mind that oxygen will often relieve nausea,** something I learned while using my hyperbaric chamber.

- **Consider alternative therapies** such as acupuncture, meditation, and creative visualization, which can help to staunch nausea. Also, it is widely known that, like our own biochemical cannabinoids, cannabis, or marijuana, helps alleviate nausea. This wasn't an option I felt comfortable with for myself, and not only because medical marijuana still isn't legal in Florida, the state where I live. Marijuana has proven to have palliative effects on pain and to relieve nausea, so I'd be remiss not to include it. Now, you can opt not to *smoke* the drug: the active chemical in marijuana, THC, is available as a synthetic in pill form—Marinol. This drug is perfectly legal, *and* often used to treat extreme anorexia associated with chemotherapy, but it can also bring relief to patients who are suffering from nausea. Unfortunately for your lungs, the drug's ability to prevent nausea—as well as the drug's ability to help prevent loss of appetite and loss of the sense of taste—is most effective when it is smoked.

Radiation

Radiation therapy is another common breast cancer treatment and it is important, in order to understand what the side effects might be and how to treat them, to understand exactly how it works. There are several ways that radiation therapy can be administered but, in the case of breast cancer, it is most common to employ *external-beam radiation therapy*, in which a form of high-energy radiation is directed at the site of the cancer from outside the body. This high-energy radiation—x-rays, or gamma rays, for example—kills cancer cells. But *how* does it kill cancer cells? It's tempting to think of the radiating beam meeting a cancer cell and simply blowing it up, or vaporizing it, as if the beam were some sci-fi video-game laser. What actually happens is that the beam kills the cancer cell by damaging its DNA, either directly or by creating free radicals within the cell that will, in turn, damage the DNA. When a cell's DNA is damaged beyond the cell's ability to repair itself, the cell stops dividing and dies. The problem with this scenario is that it is not only the cancer cells that are damaged by the radiation. Though current computer-aided technology allows doctors to target cancer cells much more accurately and precisely, normal, healthy cells in the path of the radiation beam are also unfortunately damaged. This 'collateral damage' is what causes the side effects of radiation treatment.

Now, that said—and knowing that there will be a certain amount of toxicity created in your body due to the therapy itself—radiation is often a necessary and quite successful part of cancer treatment. If radiation is part of your cancer program, you can think of it as 'the lesser of two evils' and prepare for it accordingly. Do make sure, however, that you understand the full scope of your treatment and whether or not radiation will have to be a part of that treatment before you opt for any phase of the program. For example, sometimes a woman will have the option to have a lumpectomy rather than a full mastectomy, and will choose the lumpectomy to preserve the breast. This is a perfectly acceptable course of action if it's what the patient desires, but keep in mind that when the lumpectomy is performed, the cancerous tissue may still have small seeds in the remainder of the breast tissue. Therefore, after a lumpectomy, your doctor will more than likely recommend a course of radiation to make sure that any potential 'seeds' have been killed. Being able to talk through the full scope of your treatment is another reason why it is so critical to choose doctors with whom you have a good rapport to guide you through your cancer experience.

Undergoing Radiation Therapy

Radiation therapy itself—that is, the period of time in which the radiation beam is active, is very brief, maybe ten minutes for each session. The time-consuming part of radiation is in working with your radiation technician to allow her to position your body in *exactly* the same postion for each session. Your technician will likely make a "cast" of your body before your first therapy session and will help you to position yourself in this cast for each session thereafter. When you are immobilized, she will then use a computer to direct the radiation beam to a precisely calculated spot on your body.

Sometimes other tools are used to help direct the beam—plastic casts in the shape of the patient's unique tumor, wire masks, and even temporary tattoos. Don't be hesitant to ask during each step why the doctor or technician is doing what they are doing, or employing a particular tool. Importantly, keep in mind that the breast area is very near the heart, and you will want to know if your heart is going to be involved in the radiation path. I have a friend who underwent radiation and, while she is cancer-free and very glad to have had the radiation option, she now has a prolapse of the heart valve due to radiation damage.

One other tip for you to take to heart while you're going through radiation: exercising through your treatments is empowering! Start moving as soon as you feel up to it. Walk as far and as briskly as you are able, and be sure to keep stretching to retain—or even improve!—your range of motion.

Detoxing from Radiation

So, we now know that radiation therapy can—and in almost all cases *will*—kill healthy cells as well as cancer cells by damaging their DNA or creating free radicals within in the cells. We also know that damaged DNA and free radicals are what cause cancer in the first place. And you should know as well that radiation has a half life; that is, while the amount of radiation in your body will decrease over time, it will only ever decrease by half of the amount already there, so once you have received radiation therapy you will always have a small amount of radiation in your body. Maintaining a stepped-up detoxification program while you're receiving radiation treatment, as well as after radiation is complete, is therefore paramount.

What are the best ways to detox?

● **Lymphatic massage.** We will discuss the benefits of massage in more detail in Chapter Twelve; for now, remember that our lymphatic system is designed to help move waste products and toxins out of our system and, so, a skilled lymphatic massage practitioner can help activate the lymph glands to work more quickly and efficiently to drain.

● **Acupuncture.** The flow of the lymph fluid can also be enhanced through acupuncture techniques. Your best bet in finding a good local practitioner is through recommendation, so while you could start with scouring the Internet for practitioners who are convenient to your home and within your price range, you should ask your doctor, friends, and other cancer patients and survivors about their experiences with each candidate. There are acupuncturists who specialize in cancer support, so contacting cancer support groups or organizations may be helpful.

● **Milk Thistle.** This is not a detox method, per se, rather, a support technique. The liver is the organ of the body charged with cleaning up the waste and other toxins. The toxicity of radiation puts a heavy load on your liver, then. Milk thistle, which you can find in pill or liquid form, helps to support the liver while it's doing its job.

● **Glutathione and its precursors.** This is the most powerful, natural antioxidant in your body. There are many sources out there of glutathione, and you need to find a good one because the truth is that many of them are oxidized, used up, not helpful, out of commission, unable to do their free radical scavenging job before you ever buy them and bring them home. Check the Resources section for better choices in augmenting your body's glutathione.

Skin Burns

The sun's radiation causes sunburn when we have spent too long outside on a summer's day without a good sunscreen covering our skin. Similarly, the therapy's radiation burns the skin. Sometimes pure aloe vera lotion will do the trick—and I do mean *pure*: many aloe vera lotions on the market use other ingredients along with aloe and those additional ingredients can irritate and cause further harm to already sensitive skin; the best bet if you are opting for aloe is to buy yourself a large plant and break off a stem to use the natural aloe liquid when you need burn relief. There are also many topical lotions. Your doctor can provide recommendations, or a prescription, as necessary. Remember to put any lotion on *after* your treatment as it could otherwise interfere with the radiation or exacerbate the burning side effect.

Additionally, hyperbaric therapy, as we discussed in Chapter Two, is commonly used for burn victims. The ability to soothe and help to heal radiation therapy burns and their associated discomfort or pain is another reason to avail yourself of the nearest hyperbaric chamber if you are undergoing radiation therapy.

Dry Mouth and Dry Eyes

Radiation therapy and/or chemotherapy can disrupt the flow of saliva in your mouth and interfere with the production of tears in your eyes. The problem with a lack of saliva is not simple "cotton mouth," the sort of dry mouth you can experience when you're nervous or under stress; saliva helps to regulate the bacteria in your mouth, so when you don't have enough of it, you can experience problems with your teeth and gums—cavities and gum disease. Ask your doctor to recommend an antiseptic oral rinse that will help you to continue to produce saliva during the time you are undergoing radiation, and be sure to schedule an appointment with your dentist immediately following the completion of your radiation therapy so he can assess and help you to conservatively heal any damage to your teeth or gums. As you'll read below, dental surgery in jaws that have indirectly received radiation is not lightly undertaken.

To soothe dry eye, ask your doctor to recommend a moisturizing eye drop you can use during your course of treatment. There are many of them that are preservative-free on the over-the-counter market. I recommend scheduling an appointment with your eye doctor following the completion of your radiation therapy, as this therapy has been known to cause changes in vision. You'll want to have this checked and, if you wear glasses or contacts, make certain your prescription doesn't need to be altered.

Radiation and Osteoporosis

As we've made clear, radiation doesn't impact only the part of the body at which the radiation beam is directed. It can also affect the structure of your bone marrow and bones, leading to osteoporosis, or the loss of bone density. This is more of a concern for small-boned women; those of us with larger and denser bones are less likely to have to put osteoporosis at the top of our list of concerns. In any case, I recommend having a bone density test performed prior to beginning radiation, so you have a baseline. During the period you are undergoing radiation, exercises such as brisk walking and other weight-bearing exercises (try brisk walking while carrying a one-pound weight in each hand!), will help to counter the potential for radiation-created bone loss. Then, when your radiation treatments are complete, have another bone density test so you and your doctor can determine if additional therapy to repair bone loss or prevent further loss is necessary.

Radiation and Osteonecrosis of the Jaw

Among the bones that can be impacted by radiation treatment are the *maxilla* (the upper jaw) and the *mandible* (the lower jaw). When these bones are affected, a severe disease known as osteoradionecrosis of the jaw, or ORN, can result. It can take months or even years to develop, and, boy, is it a doozie! Osteoradionecrosis literally means "death of bone due to radiation." It usually manifests after dental surgery in a jaw that has been exposed to radiation, where the blood vessels supplying the jaw have been affected—or, essentially, decreased—by radiation and there just isn't enough blood supply to heal the trauma, so the bone dies. Interestingly, the use of hyperbaric therapy as both *prophylaxis* and treatment for osteoradionecrosis of the jaw is recommended[116]—and it is not only FDA approved, and therefore a "labeled" reason to use hyperbarics, it is often a benefit covered by your insurance policy. I'm not sure this is widely known, and I'm quite certain this treatment is not widely used, so be sure to ask about *hyperbaric therapy prophylactic use* if you've had radiation therapy to your jaw and need dental work done. The unfortunate reality is that you'll probably have to advocate for yourself on this one, helping your dentist and your physician to work together on getting hyperbaric therapy prescribed and scheduled. Untreated, this disease can progress to where removal of the marrow in the bone or the removal of the bone itself is necessary.

After Radiation Therapy

Radiation therapy is normally complete after a maximum of thirty-five radiation sessions. But keep in mind that radiation is cumulative, meaning the effects will continue to get more intense *after* therapy until they level off and begin to resolve or stabilize. For example, radiation burns will likely feel worse once you leave your therapy appointment, but they

---

116 http://www.ncbi.nlm.nih.gov/pubmed/9195618.

should begin to feel better over a period of weeks. Similarly, your breast tissue will begin to change during radiation treatments. Radiated tissue tends to become coarse and dense, so the feel of your breasts will change; this change, however, will be permanent.

It's important to note as well that, should your cancer recur after radiation treatment, it is extremely rare that you will be able to use radiation as a treatment in the second round and a mastectomy will likely be your doctor's recommendation.

Surgery

Range of Motion

Several weeks before your surgery, you are going to want to start working on your range of motion, meaning how far and effortlessly you can reach your arms in all directions. That's because scar tissue wants to shrink and, if you let it, your ability to reach for a can of soup on a high kitchen shelf, or to reach behind you to close a door, will become limited. If it becomes limited, and to what degree, will depend on the work you do to address how you will allow your scar tissue to behave.

I believe that one of the most important post-operative things I did as part of my recovery was to schedule regular massage therapy sessions. These sessions were so important, in fact, and for so many myriad reasons, I have devoted an entire chapter to the benefits of massage a little later in this book. For now, let me say that massage helps your scar tissue to set up longer and with more flexibility; massage helps the scar tissue to heal the way you want it to heal.

What can you do pre-surgery to help with the way your scar tissue is going to heal? That is, how can you deal with scar tissue before you even have any? Stretch! I accomplished my stretching by way of yoga classes, working with my instructor on specific stretches and poses that would open up my chest, or stretch my chest muscles. One of the poses I did several times a day, pre-op, was to lie on my back, with a blanket roll between my shoulder blades. This lifted my chest and allowed my shoulders to stretch as wide open as possible without force, using my own body weight to gently expand their range.

I think it is also important to lift weights as part of a regular physical fitness routine. Weight bearing exercise helps to keep our muscles toned, and also to prevent osteoporosis, and it is a component of regaining our strength after we've been sick. Pre-surgery isn't a time to stop lifting weights, but you need to balance the time you spend lifting (a muscle-contracting exercise), with adequate time to stretch the muscles out after your lifting session.

What to Wear in the Hospital

Let's face it: when you are in the hospital, there is so much you are not in control of. It meant a lot to me to get back into my own pajamas as soon after surgery as I could. So pack a pair of comfortable cotton or flannel pajamas, or whatever fabric is most appealing to you to have against your skin, and make sure they button up the front so you and your nurses will have easy access to your breast and breast area.

In addition to your pajamas or the hospital gown, you will be wearing a post-op garment that functions to hold the drains and provide support. Your doctor will most likely fit you for your post-op support garment prior to the surgery itself, but what you won't be able to discern, in the short time you may try it on pre-surgery, is that it might pinch or even blister your skin when you have to wear it longer term. Mine blistered the devil out of my exquisitely sensitive skin. My mom made a very primitive wrap out of a length of flannel to go around my body underneath the garment, and the relief was tremendous. I highly recommend taking a yard or so of nice cotton flannel with you to the hospital in case you need to do the same.

Post-op you will also want some beads to wear around your neck in the shower—and I chose the least expensive, most practical and colorful option of green, gold, and purple plastic Mardi Gras beads. What in heavens name did I do that for? When you come out of surgery you will have drain tubes stitched to each of your incisions and *you will not want these drain tubes to pull.* My post-op garment had special pockets for the drains, but in the shower, I safety pinned each drain around a bead so that all the tubes didn't bunch up, and I could move without danger of them pulling when I lifted an arm or turned from the waist.

Adding to the indignities of this entire process: you'll likely have to have help showering for a day or two at least. This was a surprise for me, and as a fiercely independent kind of girl, it was hard having my husband help me bathe. Trust me: there was nothing sexy about having that angelic man try to scrub my skin with the right amount of pressure in the right places while I was still hurting from the surgery, being neurotic about the drains, having to sit down on the shower stool because I was exhausted by the whole bathing process. Those needs and feelings were gone in a week, but I did shed one or two hot angry tears of frustration in the shower in the first post-op days at home.

And, one more word about those drains: your doctor will normally remove them in his office a week to two weeks after your surgery, depending on when fluid stops accumulating in the drains. When it comes time to do this, take a pain pill because having your drains pulled is not always the most pleasant experience and, if the drain has become tangled with a nerve, its removal can be downright electric. And not in a good way! I don't care how tough you think you are—I am tough and I was so happy that a girlfriend insisted I take that pain pill. I vividly remember Ankit asking me the classic band aid removal question, "Slow or fast?" My answer was "Fast—just get it over with." It was a blanket instruction, but the removal of each of my four drains was different. The first was no big deal as it came out. The second was "special." The third was electrically shocking. The fourth was no big deal. I was glad to have the pain meds on board for the five-minute procedure, but no doubt about it, the joy of showering comfortably and independently when I got home made me feel as triumphant as the day that Rocky danced on the top step of the Philadelphia Museum of Art as he trained for his first fight.

Additionally, if you are like me, you will be happiest if you can wear your cross or other religious symbol while you are recovering. Often, however, your hospital will frown on metal jewelry and, as a breast cancer patient, you will certainly not be allowed to wear anything around your neck. My solution? I wore a wooden cross around my ankle. Worked beautifully: no one at the hospital minded at all, and I felt better.

Other Happy Hospital Tips

One of the items on your pre-surgery to-do list should be how information about how you are doing will flow to friends and family. Certainly you will neither be able to nor feel like calling anyone to update them on how you're doing, but everyone will want to know. And I really didn't even want visitors for the first two days. Rather than leave my husband, Dean, to make dozens or more phone calls, I arranged that he had to make just one phone call, to one good friend, and then that one good friend wrote up Dean's report in an e-mail and sent it to everyone on the list I supplied her with. Additionally, many cellphone apps and websites have been developed to allow friends and family to monitor your progress remotely.

When you get to the hospital on the day of your surgery, you will likely have a long wait before you are actually taken in hand and your surgery preparations will begin. To me, it is utterly ludicrous and unnecessary that a woman might need to arrive at five AM for a scheduled surgery and then sit for an hour and a half in some sterile and/or unfamiliar waiting room, until the hospital staff has time to admit her and begin her prep. Barring hospitals getting a whole lot more efficient and/or considerate in the very near future, I recommend taking a friend, reading material, and an iPod filled with music to the hospital so you will have something to do, and a way to calm your nerves while you're waiting.

Speaking of iPods, did you know that, in most cases, you need only to ask and you will be allowed to listen to music not only while you are waiting for surgery, but while you are having the surgery itself? You'll need to have a pair of ear pods—because what you're listening to can't interfere with what is going on in the operating room—but just ask your anesthesiologist to keep the pods in your ears while you are under anesthesia and music can be a part of your surgery experience for as long as your iPod's charge lasts! I loaded my iPod with beloved, peaceful music that contained 60-72 beats per minutes (to mimic the beat of the human heart), hit 'shuffle' and floated off into my surgery with joyful sounds in my ears.

In the pre-op room, one of my nurses thoughtfully placed a pillow under my head, but it was a disposable, foam OR pillow and I could not stand the smell of it, so I asked and was allowed to use my own until I was fully under anesthesia. At that point I happen to know that they take the pillow away so that your airway is in the correct position. I actually took several of my own sleeping pillows to the hospital. I think I can say with complete confidence that hospital pillows aren't very comfortable, for one thing. For another, they are usually encased in plastic protectors, and for one more thing their cases have likely been washed in stinky, heavy-duty industrial hospital detergent. Taking the pillows from your own bed to the hospital prevents these reasons for discomfort.

One post-op surprise for me was that my left elbow was very, very uncomfortable. It took me a few days to realize that it was a consequence of having had my arm strapped to the operating table for so many hours without moving. Some of the positioning in an OR is determined by what access the operating team needs for your particular procedure, but you can let the anesthesiologist know that one position feels better than another—they will try to move things around to accommodate your needs once you're asleep and the procedure is underway. Anesthesia means without pain, and those docs take that very seriously. We worked on that elbow for several weeks with post-op yoga stretching and massage.

You might also think about taking your own food to the hospital. Hospitals are supposed to be healing places, so it always shocks me anew whenever I am confronted with disgusting, inorganic hospital slop that someone thinks I'm actually going to eat. My husband and kids brought meals to me—organic, balanced, veggie-heavy, delicious meals. Until hospitals become more aware that food is the most important sort of medicine in the world, I recommend you arrange to skip the hospital tray at meal time and have some decent, whole food brought to you.

The other thing you really should bring with you, at least for the first couple of nights you are in the hospital, is another person. For me, that was my mom who, from the perspective of both mother and cancer survivor herself, simply refused to leave the hospital when visiting hours were over. I was slightly annoyed with her at first—like most of you, I am a self-sufficient sort of woman, used to giving care, not getting it, and I was rather insulted that someone—especially my own mother!—would think I couldn't get on for a few nights in the hospital on my own. Boy, was I wrong! Boy, was I glad Mom stayed!

When you are in ICU those first couple of nights, you will look like a plate of spaghetti. You may have a catheter in your bladder. You will have drains, and they will all hurt—I had two drains for my tummy tuck and one drain on each breast. You may have EKG leads, a pulse oximeter on your finger, and oxygen tubing in your nose.[117] Depending on the sort of reconstruction technique, you will have wires coming from your breasts that your doctor and nurses will use to test your new breast tissue every hour on the hour, to make sure that it is still alive and the blood supply hasn't been compromised. (If it has, you will be rushed to the OR before you have a chance to blink so they can save it. Fortunately, this is exceedingly rare, and it is one of the things that happens less and less when a surgeon does more and more microvascular surgery, so you want to find a plastic surgeon who does these procedures all of the time.)

---

117 And, let me tell you, does oxygen dry out your nose! Vaseline, or an organic Vaseline substitute, is what you'll want to keep your nose from bleeding.

Back to you as a plate of spaghetti... You will feel like the victim of an alien abduction: what isn't groggy will ache. You will not be able to reach for your own cup of water, or navigate the spaghetti to find the phone. You will need someone who can help you drink, talk on the phone, and turn over. Accept the help if it is offered to you, solicit it if it is not, and be grateful for it.

You can thank me for this tip later.

Make peace with the changes— physical, emotional, and financial— that you will be going through.

Cancer causes change. So far in this chapter we've talked a lot about the internal, emotional shift you need to make in order to empower yourself as a patient: *I come first*. But there are some concrete physical changes that are going to happen during the course of your recovery—some of them will be temporary, some permanent; some can be visible to the public, some not. All of them have the potential to affect your self-esteem, and your ability to face your on-going treatments with resolve and grace. Anticipating the changes—knowing and expecting what may come—will help you to meet the needs the changes can impose.

Short-Term Changes

The most common short-term changes you can expect as a cancer patient include fluctuations in weight, either a gain or a loss; swelling, usually of the limbs, called lymphedema; hair loss, especially if chemotherapy is part of your treatment; and changes to the skin, especially if radiation therapy is part of your treatment. None of these changes are especially pleasant— and, yes, you can count that as the understatement of the year, if you'd like. But the operative phrase to remember is that they are *short-term*: they are going to go away; you are going to address them to the best of your ability while you are going through them, *and you will get through them.*

Yes, you will come out on the other side.

Weight Gain or Loss

With breast cancer, weight fluctuations usually lean toward the—wait for it—*gaining* side of the scale. Wouldn't you know it? Often the gain is only five to ten pounds, but sometimes more, especially if chemotherapy is part of your treatment. There are many factors that contribute to this weight gain. For example, chemotherapy can bring on premature menopause, and one of the effects of menopause is to slow metabolism, so it takes more work for the body to burn calories. At the same time, the nausea, pain, and fatigue that can result from some breast cancer treatments make it less likely that you'll want to exercise while you're in treatment, and the frequently intense food cravings, particularly for carbs and sweets that chemo can trigger, might make moderating your diet a real challenge.

Add to this the impact of the ancillary drugs you may take during the course of treatment. Corticosteroids, which are used to control the nausea that can occur with chemo, and are sometimes part of the treatment themselves, can cause an increase in appetite, and they can, additionally, cause a change in body composition, redistributing muscle mass from extremities to the abdominal area, as tummy fat. Steroids, when used chronically, may also cause a loss of muscle mass and frequently result in the appearance of increased fullness in the neck, face, and abdominal areas. Hormone therapy—the use of estrogen, progesterone, and/or testosterone in treatment—can cause changes in metabolism, reduction in muscle mass, and an increase in fat mass. Tamoxifen, for example, may be a culprit in weight gain either because it causes water retention, or because it can increase the appetite.

Not all patients react to all drugs in the same way, of course. Weight loss can also happen with breast cancer, usually a result of the side effects of chemotherapy—nausea and/or loss of appetite can accompany chemo for some women. But the deck is sort of stacked in the direction of weight gain. Knowing that a few additional pounds are likely to be part of your life for a little while, however, I make this solemn recommendation: go shopping. Say what? I can help beat cancer with a spree at the mall? Yes! Stocking your closet with a few really pretty, loose dresses—mine were in cotton and linen because I went through the bulk of my cancer treatment during a Florida summer—can be a super smart move: loose clothing will help you feel comfortable during your interim weight gain, and pretty clothing can help keep you feeling attractive and confident.

The key here is to recognize that your weight is probably going to go up or down while you are healing. Prepare for how you are going to address it with a healthy diet and exercise, and understand and accept it as a temporary part of your healing process.

Sore Mouth

Sometimes chemotherapy or radiation will cause mouth sores, or oral *mucositis*, which can be very painful, even to the point where you can't swallow or eat, or it becomes uncomfortable to speak or even breathe. This can happen for a number of reasons. Both chemotherapy and radiation can weaken the body's immune system, which then allows bad bacteria, viruses, and fungi the opportunity to cause infection. Specifically in terms of chemo, it can happen because chemo drugs are designed to attack and kill fast-growing cancer cells—and the healthy cells of the mouth are generally also fast growing.

So how do you prevent and treat mouth sores? First, before you begin any chemo or radiation treatment, visit your dentist. *You will not be able to visit your dentist after you have begun your treatments because of the risk of additional infection,* so resolving any outstanding dental issues at the outset is so very important. At the very least, you will want to have your teeth cleaned before you begin cancer treatments. This is because prevention of chemo- and radiation-caused mouth sores begins with a clean mouth. While in treatment, get in the good habit of rinsing your mouth with a non-alcohol based mouthwash several times a day. Brush your teeth upon waking and before going to bed, and after every meal and snack. And, even if you have never before remembered to floss regularly, now is the time to begin to do it religiously, at least once a day.

If, in spite of these efforts, you do develop mouth sores, let's talk a little about healing, and soothing them.

First, if you smoke, here is one more reason to stop now that you have begun chemo or radiation: smoking prevents any sores you may develop during treatment from healing.

Second, eat with consideration. Have smaller meals more frequently, and take smaller bites of softer food, chewing more slowly. Avoid spicy or acidic foods, as well as alcohol, as they can further inflame an already irritated mouth, as can foods that have sharp edges like potato chips or crackers. Use a straw for drinking as it can help you to keep liquid from the sores in your mouth. Consider the temperature of your meals—foods that are room temperature will be easier on your mouth than foods that are very hot or very cold.

That said, *cold therapy*, or cryotherapy, can sometimes help reduce the risk of developing mouth sores or exacerbating existing ones, and is a rather simple procedure—it involves only swishing your mouth with ice chips for the first half an hour or so of your treatments. The cold reduces the amount of the chemotherapy drug that reaches your mouth, thus limiting the amount of damage the drug can do to the cells there.

If your mouth sores become more severe or more painful, there are medications your doctor can prescribe to offer additional relief. Palifermin is one such medication, and it works by stimulating the growth of cells on the surface of your mouth, helping them to recover more quickly from the effects of the chemotherapy drug. There are also *coating agents*, which coat the lining of your mouth, thus protecting existing sores and reducing the discomfort of eating or drinking. And *topical painkillers* can be applied directly to the sores to numb them. Your doctor might also recommend a "magic mouthwash"—a solution which can be had in commercial, pre-mixed varieties, or can be prepared by a compounding pharmacist based on your doctor's specific, individualized prescription. The basic ingredients are:

- **an antibiotic,** to kill bacteria around the sore—and if your doctor does include this as an ingredient, be vigilant about taking your probiotics to counter the effect of the antibiotic on your bowel flora;

- **an antifungal,** to kill fungal growth;

- **a corticosteroid,** to address inflammation;

- **a local anesthetic,** or antihistamine, to address and reduce discomfort;

● **an antacid** to increase the coating effect of the other ingredients over the entire lining of the mouth.

Lymphedema

Lymphedema is the swelling of an extremity—a leg or, more frequently in the case of breast cancer, an arm, shoulder, breast, chest, or hand. It is caused by the removal of lymph nodes and/ or vessels in the chest or underarm area that often occurs during cancer surgery. The lymphatic system, you'll recall, is the 'highway' by which lymphatic fluid is circulated throughout our bodies; removal of one or more lymph nodes or vessels changes the route of the lymphatic fluid, sometimes causing a build-up of the fluid in the fatty tissue beneath your skin. This build-up is what is called lymphedema.

It is difficult to predict which patient will get lymphedema, but there are some ways to try to prevent the possibility and, as science provides more advanced cancer treatment, the preventative possibilities grow. First of all, lymphedema is less possible when cancer treatment is more conservative. Additionally, you and your doctor may decide you are a candidate for a *sentinal lymph node biopsy*, which is a procedure that reduces the number of lymph nodes your surgeon needs to remove, or *axillary reverse mapping*, which is a procedure during which the lymph nodes of the arm are drained before surgery so that, if at all possible, they can be preserved rather than removed.

If you do end up with lymphedema, however, it's important to get treated early to get it under control, so knowing what symptoms to look for is key. Here they are:

- Swelling in the arm, shoulder, breast, chest or hand;

- Feeling of heaviness or fullness in the arm, shoulder, breast, chest or hand;

- Tingling sensation or an ache in the arm, shoulder, breast, chest or hand;

- Changes in the texture of the skin, e.g., tightness or hardness, or reddish discoloration;

- Less flexibility or range of motion in the nearby joints, such as the wrist, elbow, shoulder or fingers;

- Tightness or differences in the way your clothing or bra, or jewelry, such as rings or bracelets, fit;

- Rising temperature, taken with an oral thermometer, exceeding 100.5 degrees Fahrenheit, and you aren't suffering with the flu or a cold.

- Important point—if your arm, chest, breast, shoulder, hand or underarm area swells suddenly, feels hot or becomes visibly red, this could be a sign of infection or even a blood clot; in this case you should seek treatment on an emergency basis asap.

If you are diagnosed with lymphedema, you should, as we've noted, begin treatment as soon as possible. Prompt treatment will keep the swelling and any discomfort from getting worse, and prevent the possibility of infection. Treatment for lymphedema can be either of two types:

● **manual lymphatic drainage (MLD),** which is a specific type of massage that is performed along with compression therapy, gentle exercise, and skin care that the patient typically learns to perform for herself;

● **complex decongestive therapy (CDT),** which is used in cases of more severe lymphedema and involves the same sorts of therapies as MLD, but includes special bandaging. CDT is performed by a therapist who has undergone specialized training.

Treatment for lymphedema is prescribed by your doctor, and should always be administered by an experienced professional. In most cases it is covered by insurance, though you will want to check with your carrier as some policies don't cover the cost of compression garments or dressings.

Hair Loss

Hair loss is often the hardest part of chemotherapy. It is the most difficult side effect to contemplate because it is so public. As you prepare to heal, decide how you are going to handle being bald. The time-honored way to go is to wear a wig—and there are any number of salons you can go to that cater to cancer patients and stock some gorgeous wigs that really are works of art. You may decide to make a day of choosing your wig, taking your girlfriends along to try on all the various styles that are available. Will you go with a wig that replicates your own natural color and accustomed style, or will you opt for a completely different look, color and length? Remember again when Samantha was diagnosed with breast cancer on *Sex and the City*? She decided to spend a little time with hot pink hair!

While I think hot pink hair is a bold, fun move, and totally applaud bold and fun if that's your style, I opted out of even more conventional wig opportunities for several reasons. First, a side effect of chemo can be hot flashes; I knew I wanted to continue to minister to my patients as much as I was able to do so during my own treatment, and worrying through a hot flash while I was trying to examine an autistic five-year-old with a pile of synthetic hair on top of my head did not appeal to me at all. I decided I would wear colorful scarves on my head, and my friends, staff and patients began to see them as my trademark—I have a huge and beautiful collection of scarves folks gifted to me during my treatment. I actually enjoyed deciding which lovely scarf I'd put on in the mornings, and in which artful way I'd wrap it that day, and I even got one of my best cancer stories from this accessory. One of my patients, a seven-year-old boy who has made huge leaps and bounds in his recovery from autism, squinted at me as we were wrapping up his exam one day and pointed at my head. "Take that off," he commanded, letting me know that he didn't like the change. "I'll take it off, but I'm bald underneath, and it might be kind of scary," I informed him. "Take it off," he insisted. I glanced at his mom, who smiled and shrugged, so I whipped the scarf off my head. He looked at me critically for a few long seconds then said, "Put it back."

Wigs, scarves, hats, or *au naturel*—I know of one cancer patient who attended a Halloween party during her chemo as a Buddhist monk—it is important to accept that you probably will lose your hair, for a time, as you heal. Indeed, in order to own the hair loss, to be in control of it, you should choose when and how to go bald; the sensation of power in cutting your own hair, and shaving your own head, can be potent. If you decide to go that route, make sure you use an electric razor because you don't want to chance nicking your head. And remember, if you decide to go *au naturel*, be sure to wear a hat and sunscreen on your scalp when you go outdoors. One of the happy surprises about being bald was how much cooler I was! There's a lot of heat loss through the scalp, and the hot Florida summer wasn't quite so hot with no hair to deal with. I also had a bald-at-home rule. No scarves or hats at home—if you came to my house, you were going to get my bald look. It was a corollary to the no-pantyhose-at-home rule. I don't wear pantyhose inside my house, and I wasn't going to wear a scarf or hat or wig there, either.

One very practical treatment I gave myself was to rub vitamin E oil on my scalp every single day while I was bald. I'm convinced this made a huge difference as my hair grew back. Post-chemo hair can grow back with a texture like a Brillo pad; my hair grew back, and remains, baby-soft and shiny.

All of that said, there are new techniques currently being tested that may help patients keep their hair during chemotherapy treatments. One of them is the *cold cap*, which, in reality looks a bit more like a ski baklava without the portion that covers the lower face. The theory behind the cold cap is that near-to-freezing temperatures will reduce the flow of blood to the scalp which, in turn, makes it harder for the chemicals in the patient's chemo cocktail to reach, and harm, the hair follicles. Tests have, so far, been hopeful, though the FDA has yet to approve the technique.

Changes to the Skin

If you are going to have radiation therapy as part of your cancer treatment, you can expect some changes in the feel and appearance of the skin around the radiation site during, and even after, the treatment. This is because radiation therapy works by breaking down and killing cancer cells. Most radiation therapies, however efficiently they target cancer cells, also radiate—that is, *kill*—some of the healthy cells in the surrounding area, causing these areas to become red, dry, sore or sensitive to the touch, even to peel and/or blister.

There are certain areas of the breast that are more prone to these sorts of reactions than others. For example, the skin under the fold of your breast may react more significantly because it rubs against itself, or because your bra is rubbing in this area. Sensitivity may also be caused by the direction of the radiation beam: the beam is ideally positioned perpendicular to the skin, so the radiation goes *through* the skin to the targeted area; however, in the areas of the breast where the beam is parallel to the skin it 'skims' across the skin, radiating a more superficial but larger skin area.

You may also experience heightened effects in the skin in the upper corner of the radiated breast. This may be because of the angle of the beam (this is also an area where the beam may have to be directed in a parallel trajectory), but it can also be due to the fact that you like to sunbath: skin that has had significant sun exposure over many years tends to react more strongly (and/or heal less efficiently) when exposed to additional radiation.

The skin under your armpit can also be susceptible to irritation because of hair, perspiration, and the motion of the arm rubbing against radiated skin.

Other physical characteristics, as well as some treatment options, can exacerbate radiation reaction. For example, if you have large breasts, fair skin, or a history of being prone to sunburn, you might have a stronger reaction to radiation therapy. In terms of treatment options, if you are having radiation after a mastectomy and the dose is a high one, or if you are having radiation in conjunction with chemotherapy, you do have a chance of increased reaction.

Again, remember that such effects of radiation therapy are temporary—and they are also predictable *during* treatment; you and your doctor should, from visit to visit, monitor your reaction during each treatment so that she can prescribe salves or other medications to ease your discomfort, or, in more difficult cases, so you can take a break between treatments to allow your skin more time to heal.

After your radiation treatment is complete, be patient. Usually the damage from the radiation will get worse for a week or two before it begins to get better. The new skin that forms in the radiated areas may have a pearly pink or a deeply tanned look for up to six months, sometimes longer, before it returns to its natural color and texture. In rare instances, a patient may notice a small, triangular patch or patches of tiny blood vessels in the radiated areas. These are called *telangiectasias*; these don't go away on their own, but can be treated by a dermatologist with laser therapy.

Changes to the Nails

If chemo is part of your treatment, you may experience changes to your finger- and toenails. Their color may change (darken or become yellow); they may become brittle and crack more easily; light or dark lines, called Beau's lines, may appear across the width of the nail; and the nails may develop a concave appearance, called koilonychias. Infections may develop underneath the nail; nails may loosen or stop growing; and several high-dose cycles of certain chemotherapy drugs may even cause the nails to fall off. These symptoms occur, in the main, because chemo has a drying effect on the body's tissues, and while this effect is temporary, it is not usually completely preventable, and it can be painful. Here are some ways to keep nail damage and discomfort to a minimum:

- **Wear gloves** when you're engaging in activities like washing dishes and gardening;

- **Be gentle** when clipping your nails and caring for cuticles;

- **Avoid acrylic** and other artificial nails, as well as colored polishes, but do try to keep a coat of clear polish on the nails to help strengthen them;

- **If you develop Beau's lines,** cut them off as they grow beyond the nail bed;

- **As Beau's lines are caused** by a lack of iron in the diet, increase your in-take of green leafy veggies that are rich in both iron and folate, or ask your doctor about taking an iron supplement;

- **Cut out caffeine,** or cut down if you really do need that first cup in the morning, as caffeine also dries out tissue;

- **Avoid tight shoes,** or high heels that can cramp or compress the toe area;

4. **If your clinic is not among those that use cryo-therapy,** in the form of frozen gloves, to help lessen the impact of chemotherapy on the nails, ask your nurse to bring you a bowl of ice water in which to submerge your fingers during the course of each treatment.

Remember, when your treatment ends, your nails will grow back—new growth will replace the damaged tissue. Also keep in mind that fingernails grow up to three times faster than toenails, so be patient as your tootsies renew themselves at treatment's end.

Changes in Taste and Smell

It may sound silly, at first, that changes in one's ability to smell and taste are among the most common complaints for patients who are undergoing chemotherapy but, believe me, these changes are real, and no laughing matter. Our ability to appreciate the aromas of our favorite foods, and to relish the way they taste, is not part of our physiology for reasons of pleasure alone—these are built-in triggers that tell the body it needs to nourish itself. The lack of ability to smell and to taste can lead to unhealthy weight loss (to the point of malnutrition), prolonged sickness and feelings of being sick, and even decreased efficacy of the very treatments that are supposed to be helping you heal. Studies have shown that during chemotherapy taste and smell are significantly impacted for the great majority of patients.[118] Armed with this knowledge, what do we do to prepare?

First, check with your doctor regarding the specific chemotherapy drug he has prescribed for your treatment. Taxane-based drugs such as docetaxel[119] and paclitaxel[120] seem to have the most profound impact on the senses of taste and smell. Taxane-based drugs prevent the growth of cancer cells in a unique way—by rearranging the *microtubules*, a specific support structure, inside a cell, which prevents the cell from dividing in an efficient manner—and your doctor may recommend them for your unique cancer for exactly that reason. That said, check with your doctor to find out if another non-taxane-based drug might be appropriately substituted. This may seem like a preposterous sort of question to raise with your oncologist, but one of the things we don't necessarily know as lay people is that there are many regimens of chemo protocols that have been developed in different regions of the world for different cancers. Your oncologist will have protocols she's most

---

118 *http://www.ncbi.nlm.nih.gov/pubmed/19289621*.

119 Brand name Taxotere.

120 Brand name Taxol.

familiar with, but if you find something that resonates with you, it's OK to have a discussion about what protocol seems best tailored to *your* needs and desires.

Second, in so far as possible, resolve to eat appropriate quantities of nutritious foods, even when eating is not a particularly appealing activity. Measuring your food, or counting calories, can help you to make sure you're getting enough of them on a daily basis. Try adding additional herbs, spices, and other flavorings to your foods in compensation for what your senses may be lacking at this time. Of the four tastes humans sense—sweet, sour, bitter, and salty—salty is the most affected during chemo; knowing this, try not to overdo it with the salt, or use a salt-alternative that substitutes herbs and spices for the sodium chloride that is normally on our dinner tables. Recognize that, as we age, our senses tend to become less sharp in any case and, so, the older we are when we experience chemo, the greater impact the chemotherapy drugs are likely to have on our noses and tongues; for this reason, older women are going to want to be even more vigilant about regulating and monitoring diet during chemo. What was odd to me, and something my family had to become accustomed to during our weeks in what Ankit calls "Chemoland", was that I needed different seasonings to have food taste palatable. A pork chop needed some salt and some lemon. Green beans needed a sprinkle of orange juice. Be prepared to help out those four types of taste—salt, sweet, sour, and bitter—with some unusual toppings. The toppings might seem strange, but they also might make nourishing yourself when you need it most more palatable.

Finally, keep in mind that the loss of these senses is temporary; in nearly every case, they are completely recovered within three months of the end of chemotherapy.

Sleep

Imagine what would happen if you kept your coffeemaker turned on twenty-four hours a day, seven days a week—never turning it off to let it cool down, just adding water to the reservoir whenever you wanted another cup, dumping it right into the hot works, running it through the old grounds. In short order you'd have some awfully weak coffee, and, sooner rather than later you'd short the pot out and wouldn't have a coffeemaker at all!

Maybe you think this is a silly analogy for me to make—comparing the sleep of a human being and the use of a Mr. Coffee—but I am dead serious: most people would be more horrified to wake up in the morning and discover they hadn't turned their coffeemaker off the day before than they would if they woke up after less than the optimal eight hours of sleep. They would be, at the very least, dismayed about forgetting to turn off a perfectly replaceable electrical appliance, but trying to run a one-of-a-kind human body on seven, six, or even five hours of sleep a night isn't upsetting to most people; it is commonplace.

But it isn't wise.

The human body is meant to sleep though, frankly, science has yet to figure out exactly why. We know with certainty, however, what *lack* of ample sleep can do. It impairs the way your brain functions, making you groggy and grumpy and impacting your ability to remember, concentrate, and think critically. Sleep deprivation—or what is also termed *sleep debt*—has been cited as a factor in accidents and disasters from car crashes to the *Exxon Valdez* oil spill and the nuclear meltdown at Chernobyl, to the tune of 43 to 56 *billion dollars* annually.[121]

The average adult needs a minimum of six to eight hours of sleep a night. However, it is not only quantity, but also quality that matters when it comes to sleep. We need to stay asleep long enough to achieve several cycles of REM sleep, a state of deep sleep that does not even begin its first nightly cycle until we have passed through the first three stages of sleep (Light Sleep, True Sleep, and Deep Sleep), or, in other words, until we have already been asleep for seventy to ninety minutes.

The benefits of getting an adequate amount of deep, REM sleep include:

● **Improved ability** to commit new information to memory—that is, the ability to *learn*;

● **Weight control**—chronic sleep debt impacts the body's rate of metabolism, its ability to process carbohydrates, and the levels of hormones that affect appetite, thus causing the potential for weight gain;

---

121 http://web2.med.upenn.edu/uep/user_documents/dfd3.pdf.

● Heart health—increased levels of stress hormones, irregular heartbeat, and hypertension have often been caused by serious sleep disorders;

● Disease prevention, including cancer—sleep debt alters the way the body's immune system functions, including reducing the level of its natural killer cells, a type of white blood cell that plays a major role in tumor rejection.[122]

For cancer patients, then, sleep becomes important from a treatment perspective. But sleep is also critical in fighting back against a common side effect of both chemotherapy and radiation—fatigue. When I had cancer, all I really wanted to do was sleep, and I sometimes did it for sixteen to eighteen hours a day. I paid off several decades of sleep debt after my cancer diagnosis. Med school sleep deficit? Paid. Loan on sleep I took out when Dani was diagnosed with autism and I had to put myself through a new residency to learn how to treat her? Paid. Parental slumber shortage from all those nights of staying up with one of the kids when they were sick? Paid in full.

The more you can arrange to sleep while you are in treatment, the happier and, I dare say, the healthier you will be. The irony is that a lot of cancer patients—up to fully half of us— have trouble sleeping. We may be as fatigued as we have ever imagined we could ever be, but the emotional toll of coping

122 *http://www.ncbi.nlm.nih.gov/pubmed/8621064.*

with cancer, the side effects of medications, and the physical discomfort of some treatments, can make falling and staying asleep difficult for us. That's why it can be important to have a strategy for sleep.

- **Recruit your support team**, including friends and family, to let them know how important sleep will be to you during your cancer experience, and how grateful you will be for their help in facilitating it;

- **Stick to a sleep routine**, albeit one with expanded hours, even if you find you want to sleep nearly all the time;

- **Remain as physically active** as you are able during your waking hours, and try to spend some of those hours outdoors—activity and sunshine can both lead to an enhanced ability to sleep;

- **Avoid eating and drinking alcohol** for at least two hours before you want to be able to fall asleep;

- **Keep your bedroom** cool and quiet and dark, and reserve the room for sleeping only—activities such as watching TV, working on a computer or a cell phone, or taking part in a hobby can be stimulating, so you want to do those things in places other than where you sleep;

- **Put your cell phone** on airplane mode or in another room so that it's not emitting radiation near your body;

- **Decompress** and get your brain ready for sleep with activities such as reading a book or listening to soothing music.

If these suggestions don't provide a good solution in your case, you might also want to ask your doctor about taking a sleep supplement and there are many. Melatonin is a hormone that helps to induce sleep, though in too high a dose some people experience nightmares, so be conservative in how much you use at first. Also, 5HTP is known to help continue sleep, and it also helps our mood. Source matters tremendously, though, so be judicious in selecting a brand and recognize that you may need to try more than one. In a Japanese study in 2007, glycine in large doses at bedtime was found to enhance sleep quality nicely.[123] And finally, many people have significant benefit from valerian root. In very severe sleep deprivation situations, you might also ask your doctor to prescribe a drug to help you sleep.

Menopausal Symptoms/Medical Menopause

Menopause, a stage of life when menstruation ceases, happens naturally and gradually for many women when they hit their

---

123 http://dx.doi.org/10.1111/j.1479-8425.2007.00262.x.

late forties or early fifties. The body, naturally and gradually, stops producing the hormones estrogen and progesterone. For cancer patients, dealing with menopausal symptoms, and medically-induced menopause, can be an abrupt event. It can leave you coping with the classic hallmarks of midlife—hot flashes and night sweats, mood swings and memory lapses, vaginal dryness and loss of libido, fatigue and insomnia—in the midst of also coping with your cancer. For patients dealing with ovarian cancer, the removal of the ovaries coupled with pelvic-area radiation can cause abrupt and often premature menopause. For breast cancer patients, chemotherapy is usually the culprit.

Unfortunately, the traditional way of mitigating menopausal symptoms is usually not an available option for patients with either ovarian or breast cancer. This is because the traditional way has been to replace the hormones that the body is no longer manufacturing, but hormones also trigger the growth of ovarian tumors and some breast tumors: over 80% of breast cancers are hormone-receptor positive. Indeed, some cancer-fighting strategies put the hormonal responsiveness of some cancers to use in defeating them, using medications that attempt to block hormonal stimulation of the cancer cells. Eliminating the production of hormones, however, can serve to increase the menopausal symptoms the patient may experience.

Bio-identical hormones are sometimes thought of in this context as 'safe' alternatives to traditional hormones because they are plant-based versus manufactured from the urine of pregnant horses. But understand that the effect they have on cancer cells is the same—both traditional and bio-identical hormones stimulate growth—so bio-identical hormones are not a good alternative therapy for breast cancer patients who are trying to relieve menopausal symptoms.

So, then, what is the breast cancer patient who is suffering menopausal symptoms to do? There are some avenues for relief and, as usual, a generally healthy lifestyle is one of the most effective. Your best line of defense is regular exercise, quality supplements, especially calcium and vitamin D to combat the onset of osteoporosis that menopause can provoke, and a good diet that limits artificial stimulants and depressants such as caffeine, sugar and alcohol.

Additionally, selective serotonin uptake inhibitors, or SSRIs, may be helpful in alleviating menopausal symptoms. Best known as antidepressants, they work by balancing the brain's level of serotonin, a neurotransmitter that helps brain cells communicate with each other. This class of drug has also proved effective in decreasing hot flashes, and there seem to be, to date, no contraindications for breast cancer patients. The natural alternative to SSRIs is the 5HTP I mentioned earlier, in the sleep discussion. Although there isn't a lot of research available (funding research is hard to do!), I have often found that 5HTP can be helpful to folks who want to avoid prescription alternatives. Ask your doctor about other, non-hormonal drugs, such as Gabapentin, a medicine that has been used for seizures. The supplement that is most similar to Gabapentin is GABA, and while studies have supposedly shown that GABA doesn't cross the blood/brain barrier, we have used it pretty regularly in autism and families have seen a reduction in anxiety and seizure duration, and an increase in speech and that coveted sense of calm. Clonidine, used as an antihypertensive, has been deployed successfully to reduce menopausal symptoms, probably because its mechanism of action is to block some of the body's sympathetic fight-or-flight responses. Low-dose estrogen may be used locally, in the form of cream, suppositories, or vaginal ring inserts, to treat vaginal dryness or atrophic vaginitis wherein the vaginal skin becomes painfully thin. The decision to use something topically and locally rather than systemically, if you have an estrogen-positive cancer, will be one you'll have to consider very carefully.

Fertility/Family Planning and Nursing

About 5% of breast cancer cases in the US are diagnosed in women who are under forty years of age[124]—a seemingly small percentage until you put together these two facts: treatment for breast cancer, specifically both chemotherapy and tamoxifen, can cause either temporary or permanent infertility, and some of that small percentage of women under forty who are diagnosed with breast cancer are still hoping to have children, or to have more children. But a study presented at the 2009 American Society of Clinical Oncology (ASCO) Annual Meeting, found that oncologists were not giving their breast cancer

---

124 http://ww5.komen.org/BreastCancer/YoungWomenandBreastCancer.html.

patients enough information about fertility issues:[125] only 36% were familiar with their organization's own guidelines on fertility counseling and management for breast cancer patients, and fewer than 25% gave patients printed information about treatment-related fertility issues or referred them to fertility specialists. We can safely say that fertility-related issues are often overlooked—and, perhaps, rightly so from the perspective of life-saving measures that are appropriate for the patient herself. But approaching a cancer diagnosis with the intent of beating it—as we all do, of course—means that we necessarily have to consider life, and the quality of the lives we want to create, on the other side of the victory. So here are a few basic facts to explore if you wish to consider childbearing following your victory over cancer.

- **Chemotherapy is likely** to cause permanent loss of one's period, though certain chemotherapy drugs or combinations of drugs are more likely than others to cause this loss;

- **Chemotherapy can damage** some of the eggs that are stored in the ovaries, though the type of drug that is administered, and the dosage of it can be significant—alkylating drugs and nitrosoureas, for example, are more likely to cause infertility than other chemo drugs;

---

125 *http://www.breastcancer.org/research-news/20090602.*

- **Tamoxifen may cause** temporary, though sometimes permanent, menopause;

- **Periods may return** after the completion of treatment, but this does not automatically mean fertility has returned as eggs might have been damaged during therapy;

- **Women who are older** when they begin treatment for breast cancer are less likely to have their periods return when treatment is complete;

- **Chemotherapy and Tamoxifen** tend to accelerate the onset of natural menopause by as much as five years;

- **Some women,** depending on the drug used and its dosage, will remain fertile during chemotherapy but should not become pregnant while undergoing treatment because of the danger of birth defects.

Given these stark concerns, what should you do when you're diagnosed with breast cancer but would like to do the best you can to preserve your fertility options? Add a fertility specialist to your healing team. Storing embryos for implantation after treatment is complete is one option, as is storing unfertilized eggs, though this method is more experimental. There are also drugs that can "shut down" the ovaries during chemotherapy and, in doing so, theoretically protect them from the effects of the chemo drug. Such drugs, like goserelin, sold under the brand name Zoladex, are hormone-based, and their use should be considered experimental.

Other options exist, of course. Surrogacy, while potentially complicated, might be perfect for some people. Adoption in its myriad forms is no longer off the table for someone who has survived cancer and may be another viable approach. Thinking creatively and brainstorming out loud can help solve what might otherwise feel like an insurmountable problem.

Craving for Intimacy Partnered with Loss of Libido

Breast cancer changes your body. Surgeries, such as lumpectomies or mastectomies, can change the body's contours; treatments like chemotherapy and radiation can sap the body's energy, including libido, or sexual energy. Even when the libido isn't directly impacted or can be coaxed into an appearance, chemically-induced vaginal dryness can be a challenge.

Paradoxically, breast cancer can trigger a need or craving for intimacy, though, at least temporarily, it can change the way you experience or want to experience intimacy with your partner. Your gynecologist may be able to help with some of the physical challenges; the use of a water-based lubricant such as K-Y Jelly may be helpful as well. Most beneficial of all, however, is to make sure the lines of communication are open between yourself and your partner, and that you are each honestly communicating your needs to the other. While physical intimacy may be an on-going challenge when you are going through and healing from breast cancer treatment, and require loving compromises, it can also be an opportunity to grow in emotional intimacy. My husband and I had to live through the challenge of autism before we had to live through the challenge of cancer, and we joke that it was actually very good for our marriage as we really had to hone our communication skills rather than get lazy about them. Breast cancer, as I've counseled other couples facing the challenge, requires intense disinhibition when communicating—we have to be willing to talk about details and mechanics, things that can feel awkward to most of us. But that releasing of inhibitions, coupled with a whole lot of creative thinking, can make intimacy something different, something brand new and satisfying.

Long-Term and Permanent Changes

Let's talk for a moment about the way breast cancer changes the contours of our bodies—and let's get as real as it is possible to get while we do. Breast cancer changes your body. It will never be the same after your breast cancer experience. You will likely come out of the experience with scars—a port scar, scars from your mastectomy and/or reconstruction. The question is not *if* you will have scars, but how many scars will you have, where will they be located, how will they limit the range of your motion, and how will they change your wardrobe choices?

Although your body will never be the same again, there are two things that you can count on to be true.

First, since an external prosthesis is a very rare thing these days, an asymmetrical outcome, or the need for special gear like a mastectomy swimsuit, is highly unusual. This is because the techniques used in performing mastectomies and doing reconstruction change very rapidly, and with each change, the technique is improved. For example, as of this writing, I haven't been asked to show the outcome of my surgery for over two years; this is because, in the little over three years since my surgery, techniques have improved so much (and, in my case, my reconstruction surgeon has trained the general surgeons with whom he works so well to perform mastectomies in ways that will provide the best reconstructive outcome), there are now even more natural outcomes out there than mine—and mine are outstanding! Having a greater influence on your cosmetic outcome is why I feel so strongly about seeing and choosing a plastic surgeon first as you build your cancer treating team. This is not a politically correct recommendation in the medical world, but I do feel strongly about it.

Second, keep in mind that the vast, overwhelming majority of the rest of the people in the world will never know you are a breast cancer survivor. When your hair grows back and your surgery is complete, you no longer look so pale and you've got your strength back, it is beyond difficult to tell the breast cancer survivor from someone who has never had the experience... *with this exception*: there is a richness of experience, a 'steel magnolia' quality about those of us who have been on the breast cancer journey, and somehow we recognize this about each other. We are members of an exclusive club and, while

I have met women who remain bitter and angry through the process, most of us grab hold of the growth opportunity that cancer presents, and part of being forever changed by cancer means that we are forever changed for the better.

Emotional Changes

The emotional stages you will go through following your diagnosis of breast cancer are likely to mirror the stages of grief: denial, anger, bargaining, depression, and acceptance. In denial, you are in shock, numb, overwhelmed—but, hopefully, this phase is a brief one. While a period of denial is frequently necessary—it enables you to pace how you deal with grief, absorbing as much as you can handle in small portions—it also represents a period in which you relinquish control over your body and the treatment of what is ailing it.

You may also get angry with your body, feel betrayed by it and/or by a new sense of its vulnerability, or the fragility of life in general. You may do a little bargaining, with yourself, your doctors, or even with God—'If this test turns out to be negative, I promise I will never again do this other bad thing' though any example of what that bad thing might be would be fruitless because most often you're trying to bargain apples for oranges: there is nothing as valuable as your health that you can bargain away.

Be gentle with yourself—allow yourself the time and space you need to work through the shock, the anger. By all means, if you get stuck in depression, talk to your doctor—ask if the short-term use of an anti-depressant might be helpful and/or appropriate, or if she can recommend a counselor who is experienced in helping cancer patients work through their grief. The goal is to move steadily through the grief process toward acceptance, the place where you make peace with your diagnosis, because it is from that place of peace, firmly grounded in the reality of what lies ahead, that you can most effectively begin to fight back.

Relationship Changes

The changes in the relationships you share with the people in your life can be among the most difficult emotional changes that come with having cancer. I had a patient who was scheduled to see me after months of waiting. When she heard I had breast cancer, she cancelled the appointment. Three years later she sat down in the exam room and told me why she had done it. I smiled a 'steel magnolia' smile and finished the phrase she started saying: "Because you were afraid I would die." She nodded yes. Some of the football players I take care of ran for the hills. I noticed that even among the people who stood by me, some of them looked at me, at least from time to time, as if I was going to die.

Telling my patients and reassuring them was draining, but every time I did it, I talked about the elephant in the room—death. And talking frankly with people I love gave me lasting commitment to the battle, and immeasurable peace as a result. At the end of a visit with one of my favorite teenaged patients, he quickly left and walked out to the car. I had a puzzled look on my face and his mother said to me that he was really struggling with my having cancer. I was incredulous. "Why? Does he think I'm going to die?" As his mom nodded with tears in her eyes, I ran out to the parking lot, calling back over my shoulder, "Well, I'm not!" I caught up to my patient at the back of his car, calling to him, "Dude. Mom says you're freaking that I might die?" He nodded and looked down at the ground. "Well I'm not. Going. To. Die. Period." He looked straight into my eyes, whispering, "Promise?" "Promise," I answered. That very direct approach helped me tremendously to move to acceptance of my cancer and to get ready for the battle for my health.

Some people stood with me, some could not—I had and have no energy to judge anyone based on how they coped or did not cope with my cancer. I'm much more of a count-your-blessings kind of person. What I can do is tell you that often I felt as if I was spending more time consoling other people about my cancer than I was spending consoling me—and that ultimately I decided, while the consolation could be draining, cancer was proving to be just another amazing opportunity to grow—grow myself, and grow my relationships. And that, ultimately, was an empowering process.

Financial Changes

Having breast cancer is expensive. The financial stress a major disease can have on the family budget can also cause emotional stress in the household—and we've already discussed at length how unhealthy emotional stress can be. So take the time to reduce the budgetary stress to the best of your ability.

Contact your insurance provider to review your coverage so that you understand your policy's terms and what your responsibilities will be. Revise your budget to include breast cancer-specific costs that might not be covered by your insurer—items such as copayments, insurance premiums, medication copayments, supplements you may choose to use, and perhaps even compression bandages. If you are, as I was, working at the time of your diagnosis, check into the federal laws that protect your job, and your health insurance. Contact your company's Human Resources department so you are sure you know the company's sick leave policy. Keep good records of your treatments, their costs, and when and who paid for each one or portion of one. These records don't have to be elaborate, just thorough—I kept mine under one of the tabs in the folder I created to house my pathology report. Clear records will likely be helpful in preventing any disputes with management in the future, and at tax season you may be able to benefit from medical tax deductions.

Put together a Super Bowl-caliber healing team.

There are a lot of things in life you can do alone, and a lot of things you *want* to do alone. I can, should the circumstances demand it, file my own quarterly taxes. I (frequently) want to take my evening walk by myself because it is a quiet time for me to clear my head, release some of the day's stress, pray.

Cancer is a thing you cannot and do not want to do alone.

In this section we're going to talk about the different people, or groups of people, you need to enlist as part of your core cancer-fighting team.

Breast Care Coordinator

Your Breast Care Coordinator is your resource person. Beating breast cancer is a multi-disciplinary adventure. It requires the talents of a range of medical experts and your Breast Care Coordinator will help you to coordinate appointments and share information with these various experts.

Before I left the hospital following my biopsy, my Breast Care Coordinator, Peggy Neville, BSN, had everything written on paper for me—all the phone numbers for the doctors we talked about, their addresses, what I needed to do, what she had already done, and a reminder to pick up my films before going up to see my general surgeon. Peggy came to my surgical appointments and kept in touch by email or phone all the way through my treatment. She wasn't afraid of the process, and she celebrated the good things—I still remember the wonder in her voice when she commented on how soft my new hair was when it grew back.

Breast Radiologist

Breast Radiologists are medical doctors who specialize in targeted and minimally invasive medical procedures and diagnostics that are guided by imaging technologies. Mine was Mary Alderman, MD, a gifted radiologist and a friend.

Mary talked me through my breast biopsy and, when lymph nodes were questionable on the breast MRI, she biopsied those. Because she knew and respected my integrative medicine approach, she helped me find an oncologist who wasn't going to yell at me or fire me over my use of antioxidants and hyperbarics. She and I talked about treatment options all the way through the procedure, and she was there for my sentinel node biopsy on the day of surgery.

Integrative Medicine Family Practitioner

'Integrative medicine' is a term often used interchangeably with 'functional medicine'—they both refer to an approach to medicine that addresses not the disease, but the person who has the disease, and focuses on treating the body, mind, and spirit as a whole rather than separate or disconnected entities. Stephanie Cave, MD, an Integrative Medicine Family Practitioner, was the first person I called after my biopsy.

A guru in my field of autism, Stephanie also works with folks who have cancer, often those who are end-stage, when everyone else says, "There's nothing more I can do for you." I was already familiar with what Stephanie was likely to tell me to do because she had worked with a dear friend who had recently survived simultaneous prostate cancer and chronic lymphocytic leukemia. I wasn't waiting until I was end-stage to use an approach I knew would be tremendously helpful. Stephanie got my diet in order, told me what supplements to take orally, and designed the IVs that we still infuse twice weekly—they are rich in vitamins and minerals with antioxidants and really helped to get me back on my feet more quickly and with better energy. She also made me aware of the influence of electromagnetic fields on my health, and taught me how to decrease that influence.

Oncologist

An oncologist is a doctor who specializes in the treatment of cancer; a *medical oncologist* is a doctor who specializes in treating cancer with chemotherapy while a *radiation oncologist* is a doctor who specializes in treating cancer with radiation therapy. I trusted Dr. Mary Alderman and Dr. Katherine Pearson (another radiologist at the Women's Breast Center who understood and endorsed Integrative Medicine approaches to disease) to present my case at weekly "Tumor Board," where each newly diagnosed case is discussed, and pick an oncologist for me. Why did I need to approach choosing an oncologist with delicacy? Chemotherapy was the recommended course of therapy for me and most mainstream oncology folks will tell you that antioxidants are bad for you when you're having chemo, and that hyperbarics will make your tumor grow. I could not disagree more. I knew that I would pursue an integrative approach that included use of both antioxidants and hyperbarics, I would not lie about it, and I didn't want to fight about it with my own doctor. Unni Thomas, MD, was, at the very least, not opposed to an integrative approach, so he was the oncologist I settled on. He listened quietly to the rationales and science behind the functional medicine aspects I used to enhance my traditional treatments, was occasionally intrigued, and was always kind and caring.

Breast/General Surgeon

Your general surgeon is the doctor who will be responsible for removing the cancerous tissue from your body. It is important for you to feel confident in your surgeon's abilities and comfortable talking with him/her about the procedure. Thanks to the Internet, it is now fairly easy to read about a surgeon's background and expertise, and even get former patient's comments.

In choosing my general surgeon, there were several qualifications that were top of mind. First, the doctor I chose, Gary Bowers, MD, was famous for his fierce perfectionism in the OR. Second, he respected my integrative approach to dealing with my cancer. Third, he was in regular communication with Dr. Thomas, my oncologist, to coordinate my treatment through the course of my therapy.

One last thing I think is extremely important is that Dr. Bowers is a *thinking surgeon*. I wanted to do my mastectomies and my reconstruction surgery as one procedure, versus doing them separately as is more traditional. He listened to my desires, though he couldn't believe I wanted to do everything at once, committing to at least a twelve-hour surgery. His concerns? That reconstruction complications would slow down any chemo schedule I might have to be on after surgery, or that reconstruction might be compromised if I had to have radiation following surgery. I, on the other hand, wanted to be anesthetized once, not twice. I didn't want to deal with expanders and prostheses—options we'll discuss in more detail in Chapter Nine—which I would not have to do if I exercised the cutting-edge reconstruction option that was available to me. I didn't want to have to recover my body twice. And I knew that with an integrated approach to cancer and surgery, I would knock the entire team sideways with how quickly I healed and recovered. Dr. Bowers and I thought this through together, and created compromises that allowed him to be confident he was doing his job, and me to feel comfortable that my wishes were being met.

Reconstructive Surgeon

Reconstructive surgeons use surgery to restore the form and/or the function of the body. After a tour of the Internet and researching breast reconstructive possibilities, I knew that my plastic surgeon would be the member of my healing team of doctors with whom I'd have the longest standing relationship—although at the time I did not know my reconstructive surgeon would be Ankit Desai, MD or that we'd end up writing this book together and forming a professional partnership. The reason I knew at the outset that my reconstructive surgeon and I were going to have a long relationship was because, as I explained in an earlier chapter, I was going to work through my cancer with the end result in mind: the cancer would be gone from my body and I would have a fabulous reconstructive outcome. Importantly, my reconstructive surgeon was going to have to step into the OR immediately after my general surgeon finished excising my cancerous tissue—and the general surgeon would have to excise the cancer in a manner that left remaining tissues intact as the reconstructive surgeon required them to be. In this light, let me repeat here my advice that might sound, at first hearing, counterintuitive: choose your reconstructive surgeon before you choose your general surgeon. Here's why: when you and your reconstructive surgeon have discussed your unique cancer in detail, and determined the reconstructive option that is most appropriate for both the physical characteristics of your particular cancer and your reconstructive desires, the reconstructive surgeon will be able to recommend a general surgeon who is most capable of performing the techniques that are most likely to result in the desired reconstructive outcome.

Personal Supporters

Enlist everyone in your recovery.

Cancer is not something you can go through alone, as we have said, so I do not understand why it is a thing that some people still keep secret. I told everyone. I was straight-forward in telling peole how they could help me and I drew strength from each and every supporter.

I needed my children to understand that things smelled lousy to me during chemo and that the Sharpies they used to do art were just one of the smells I could not abide at this time—that I would not gag when I walked into their rooms if they limited their use of Sharpies to their father's office. I needed my husband to understand that once I was asleep, if I were to remain that way, nothing, not even him trying to get quietly into the bed, could disturb me—and I was deeply touched when he went above and beyond to meet my needs by placing an air mattress next to our bed and sleeping on that on nights that he went to bed later than I did.

I was going to continue to work as much as possible during my treatment, and in order to do so I needed my staff to guard me fiercely—to confirm appointments and reschedule anyone who was sick, to keep my appointments to a maximum of four hours per day, to schedule my infusions and hyperbaric sessions in between patients so I could keep up my energy.

I told all of the communities of which I am a part and they all rallied around my family. The autism community prepared meals in the post-op period, which was huge because my children eat a very specialized diet that the usual church groups have a harder time preparing. My son's Boy Scout troop rallied around him and helped out whenever our family needed something they could provide. My prayer group astonished me—I was shocked at how quickly and significantly the prayers started when I invited them. The power of the Internet to put a spiritual safety net together in a couple of days is amazing. The cards poured in and we used them to paper the hallway of my office. I looked at them as I walked up and down it, and the loving energy bathed me whenever I worked.

Pets

Those of us who love animals have an intuitive understanding of how good our pets are for our health. We can *feel* our blood pressure lessening when we scoop up our cat or scratch our dog's ears or ride our horse at the end of a hard day. We don't need a quarter century of scientific studies to back us up—but the studies are out there and we'll get to them shortly, but first I want to tell you about my dog, Flux.

Well, actually, Flux is my daughter's service dog, a big Golden Retriever whose joy in life is—like most dogs—to spend time with, and please, his people. Though Flux came into our household at exactly the same time as I was first diagnosed with cancer—and though one of my first considerations at the time was that I would never have enough energy to deal with undergoing cancer treatment *and* training a new puppy— I thank God that she was part of our family during my cancer experience.

Here are just a few examples of the proven benefits of pets:

- **Levels of the stress hormone cortisol** can be reduced with as little as five minutes of interaction with a dog;[126]

- **Levels of dopamine** and the endorphins that are associated with feelings of well-being are increased after only thirty minutes of interaction with a dog;[127]

- **Fewer allergies** and incidences of asthma for children who grow up with pets in their households than for children who are not exposed to animals at an early age;[128]

- **Fewer visits to the doctor** every year for older people who own pets than for non-pet-owners.[129]

- **Indeed, even watching fish** in an aquarium can decrease one's pulse rate and muscle tension![130]

---

126 "Measuring stress and immune response in healthcare professionals following interaction with a therapy dog: pilot study," S. Barker, J. Knisely, N. McCain, A. Best, Psychological Reports, 96:713-729 (2005).

127 "Animal-assisted therapy—magic or medicine?" J. Odendaal, Psychosomatic Research, 49(4):275-280 (2000).

128 "Effects of dog ownership and genotype on immune development and atopy in infancy," J. Gern, C. Reasdon, S. Hoffjan, Z. Li, K. Rogberg, W. Neaville, K. Carlson-Dakes, K. Alder, R. Hamilton, E. Anderson, S. Gilbertson White, C. Tisler, D. Dasilva, K. Anklam, L. Mikus, L. Rosenthal, C. Ober, R. Gangon, R. Lemanske, Clinical Immunology, 113(2):307-314 (2004).

129 "Stressful life events and use of physicians' services among the elderly: the moderating role of pet ownership," J.M. Siegel, Personal Social Psychology, 58:1081-1086 (1990).

130 "Effects of watching aquariums on elders' stress," M.M. DeSchriver, C.C. Riddick, Anthrozoos 4(1):44-48 (1990).

Why? How do our animal companions manage to be so very, very good for us? What cancer-specific advantages did I gain as a dog owner?

1. Animal companions offer unconditional love *and the most uncomplicated companionship*. I knew my husband and my kids would love me through my cancer—bald head, dark eye circles, zero energy and all. And I never once felt the need to try to 'look good' for them so they would love me more, but what I did feel on an almost regular basis was the desire to look as good as I could for them so that they would *worry less*. Sometimes, for example, I felt the need to slap a smile on my face when my kids were around, even though the effort was positively Sisyphean. You never have to worry about smiling for a cat or a dog; you never have to worry about an animal worrying about you—if you're in a down place, they don't require a mask or an explanation, they simply adjust their mood to fit yours. Also, they never get their feelings hurt if you don't want to talk, and they never, ever offer unsolicited advice.

2. Even when you're sick, animals will allow you to nurture them. Cats, dogs, fish, hamsters and horses: they all need to be cared for—they need to be, for example, fed on a certain daily schedule. Now, like most cancer patients, I gratefully abdicated kitchen duty to my husband, my mother, and my generous friends and neighbors during

my treatment period; cooking a meal for the whole family was simply beyond my capacity at the time. But what I could still do was make sure Flux's dish was filled at dinnertime. Everybody else in my life, including my patients, was making an extra effort to nurture me (or, if not me directly, then themselves) at that critical time—efforts that were appropriate and appreciated; but Flux had no scruples about allowing me to continue to nurture her while I was sick. The routine of it, the responsibility of it, the simple *pleasure* of it, were reminders of what my life was like before cancer, and what it was going to be like again after it.

3. Dogs (as opposed to cats and hamsters, which I also love, so no need for cat-lovers to take offense!) *need to be walked*. Flux is a big breed and she needs to be walked for at least a mile or two every day. This need could not have meshed more perfectly with my need for exercise. Taking Flux on her daily walks as often as I could got me feeling so strong that, indeed, on rainy days, or on days when Flux was off at an event with Dani and not available as a walking companion, I layered in gentle work on an elliptical. Post-cancer, I've stayed religious about exercising at least five to six days a week. We'll discuss in more depth the importance of exercise in treating cancer in Chapter Ten; for now, let me just say that it makes a tremendous difference in how I feel, both physically and mentally, and—for us breast cancer patients—it is critical to getting and keeping the estrogen-producing fat off our bodies.

As you can tell, I firmly believe in the power of animals to help their human companions heal. But there are circumstances in which a healthcare provider might recommend that a person give up her animal companion or companions, and having cancer can be one of those times. The concern in these cases is likely to be *zoonoses*, or diseases that have been known to be transmitted between humans and animals. Having to give up a beloved companion, however, can also have grave detrimental health effects, and so I believe there are very few instances where this severe step is actually necessary. If your doctor advises such a step, I would require that he or she be very specific about the reason for it. Even then I would ask if the separation had to be permanent, and I would likely seek out a second opinion before I set about finding a good new permanent or foster home for my animal.

Set positive, post-cancer goals.

This part of the assignment is almost self-explanatory: think about what you are going to do *after* you beat cancer. Now, some of you might groan at just the idea of this advice, but I am a big proponent of *thinking beyond the cancer*. Why?

When I was a student, if all I had focused on was the physical and mental exhaustion that resulted from the gauntlet of med school, I would never have graduated. I needed to have a goal, something to focus on to get through the grueling ordeal. I was going to be a pediatrician so I focused on my future patients: smiling children, happy parents. These were the images that buoyed me through thirty-six-hour shifts and helped me to earn my medical degree.

When it came time to earn my degree in cancer survival, I relied on the same, tested and true strategy: find a goal or, better yet, a few goals! The ones I focused on to get me through cancer treatment touched on every aspect of my life.

● **One of the first things** I knew I wanted to do for the new, post-cancer me was to buy new bras. My new tatas were a reason to completely clean out my lingerie drawer, toss out what no longer fit and upgrade! Before cancer I was never comfortable spending money on myself, especially on something as private and unseen as underwear. But cancer is truly one of the most acute 'I'm worth it' moments a woman can ever have. My new *girls* are now embraced every day by the comfortable, supportive, well-fitting bras they deserve.

● **I wanted to miss** as little work as possible. I didn't want to let my patients down, and I didn't want to miss them or their progress either. My solution was to stay working for the duration, but to cut back to just a few hours a day, and to take Fridays off completely. Indeed, one of the ways in which I continue to care for myself—to implement that I-come-first thinking—is that to this day I still take every Friday off. I took them and I never gave them back—and I don't ever intend to.

● **Taking Fridays off** allowed me to better fulfill another post-cancer goal, and that was to spend more time with my children, doing the things as a family that I knew had better be done now, while they were young, before they no longer got a thrill out of going to Disney World with Mom and Dad, and tromping around Greece with friends became much more attractive than doing so with the parents.

● **I had a fitness goal**: to continue to lose weight and get in shape. Pre-cancer, my physical fitness parameters began and ended with 'can I get out of bed and go to the office and see patients.' Post-cancer they are so much broader! Can I finish a five-mile hike with my son? Can I finish a marathon bathing suit shopping spree with my daughter? Can I have a fulfilling and productive day seeing patients and still have the energy to go to choir practice and sing my heart out? And, after that, can I meet my husband for dinner and have a truly romantic evening rather than falling asleep over my pork chop? I can, without hesitation, currently answer 'yes' to all of these questions, so it is time, once again, for my parameters to grow.

You see, this is my ultimate goal: to grow. To get younger every day, to celebrate *backwards* birthdays. Since I've had cancer, and have begun taking better care of myself, I have more energy to do more things than I did before I got sick. I weigh less. My hair is less gray—yes, *less* gray; just ask my hair stylist who's been with me through it all. I feel as if I'm forty, not fifty. The only thing about my body that is not better than it was before surgery is that my delicious, voluptuous, never-need-mascara eyelashes did not return with the same vigor as my hair; they are just regular old lashes these days. The rest of me, including my get-up-and-go, is all better. When you wake up in the morning feeling at least ten years younger than you really are, then waving that organic, toxin-free mascara wand a few times feels like a very small price to pay indeed.

9

Mastectomy and Breast Reconstruction

It isn't that breast reconstruction techniques, like treatments for breast cancer itself, have come such a long way in the last twenty years—it's that they've come such a long, long, long way in the last three to five years. To say nothing of how far they've come in the last three to five months.

Ankit

Before I became a dad and happily surrendered the trunk space in my car to the transport of baby gear, what it was filled with was sports gear—golf clubs, running shoes, and basketballs. I loved going to the gym on Wednesday night to play a game of pick-up basketball. It's one of my favorite ways to exercise, and to decompress. Now, while I know that at the end of the game I'm going to feel good both physically and mentally, what I never know is how the game is going to begin. How many others are going to show up and feel like playing some hoops? What kind of shape are they in? What is each player's skill level? What stressors in his home or business life might affect his game? These are just some of the variables that can determine how the teams on any given Wednesday night might shake out, and what strategy a particular team with a particular assembly of players might adopt to win. All of the players know this: when we go into the gym, we need to remain flexible and adapt our play to the circumstances of that unique day.

That is the same way you and your doctors will approach your cancer treatment: you will need to adapt to the circumstances of your particular cancer. As Julie and I have said before in this book, there are variables specific to each woman's diagnosis that affect the progress of her treatment:

- **Where is the cancer located within the breast?**

- **Are the lymph nodes involved?**

- **How big is the tumor?**

- **What stage is the cancer in** and how aggressive are the cancer cells?

- **How old is the patient?**

- **Does the patient have children already,** or does she want to try to preserve her ability to have children in her post-cancer life?

These are just some of the factors to take into consideration. Think of it this way—every woman's cancer treatment is a custom-made plan.

In this chapter I'm going to talk about the variables you'll need to take into consideration when it comes to the surgical portion of your breast cancer treatment—lumpectomy, mastectomy and/or breast reconstruction. Before we do that, however, I want to make you aware of two overarching principles, or touchstones that can help you approach this aspect of your recovery with confidence and realism.

The first of these touchstones is that, while I am going to be as comprehensive as is possible *as of this writing* in covering the options that are currently available regarding breast reconstruction, *reading a book is never a substitute for sitting down with a knowledgeable doctor to discuss the path you will take as you contemplate your breast cancer surgery.* Please approach the information I provide in this chapter as the guidelines you will use when discussing your particular breast cancer situation with your doctor or doctors.

Why this specific guideline? Well, beyond the factors that are unique to your life and your breast cancer and how they will inform your choices, there is the simple fact that the technology around breast reconstruction and the techniques that are available to reconstructive surgeons are always changing. They are getting better by the year, the month, and sometimes the week.[131] Because of today's less radical treatment for breast cancer, and the rapid development of ever newer reconstructive techniques, plastic surgeons can create more natural feeling and aesthetically pleasing breasts.

That said, I offer my second guideline for your reconstruction plan and that is, *no matter how advanced the technologies*

---

131 I update the information on my web site, *http://www.plasticsurgeryjacksonville.com* as frequently as I am comfortable that new technologies and techniques provide my patients with good or improved outcomes; you are welcome to check there for updated information. Additionally, look for updated editions of *Breast Cancer: Start Here.*

and techniques plastic surgeons can now employ to reconstruct the female breast after mastectomy, or mastectomies, your breast will be different after your surgery.

I had one young patient come into my office after her diagnosis of breast cancer and she told me, tearfully, that she didn't care what I did, she wanted her breasts to look and feel and experience the same sensations after surgery as they did prior to her operations. I completely understood where she was coming from—but I also knew that she was in the 'denial' stage of grief. The fact is that breast cancer is a life-changing event, and part of that change, when treatment involves surgery and reconstruction, is that your breasts will be different after the surgery than they are before it. For example, though there are techniques surgeons can use to minimize scarring—and though there are steps that patients can take to further reduce the appearance of scarring, and time itself reduces the appearance of scars—the fact remains that there will be a certain amount of scarring after your surgery. As another example, if your reconstruction surgery cannot include nipple-sparing techniques due to the size or location of your cancer, your new nipples, fashioned from, for instance, tummy tissue, will not have the same level of sensitivity to which you have been accustomed. Julie's surgery was a DIEP Flap, a procedure we'll discuss in more detail in a few pages; for now, what you need to know is that the procedure removes tummy skin and fat, creating the new breast or breasts from this tissue. Julie, who is the personification of positive thinking, replied to my pre-surgery cautions, "Yes, but I'm also getting a tummy tuck!"

Among the changes that breast cancer brings are changes in the way your breasts look. Talk to your doctor about the changes you can expect from your own surgery. Ask where your scars will be located. Ask what you can anticipate in terms of sensation in your breasts and in your nipples. Ask about any pain you might experience in your breasts and, if applicable, in any donor sites (sites on your body from which muscle or tissue is donated to form your new breast or breasts). Importantly, ask to see "before and after" photos of similar procedures your surgeon has performed. Plastic surgeons don't take these sorts of photos only to demonstrate their skills, but to help you realistically visualize the outcome of your own reconstruction procedure.

Mastectomy

Mastectomy is the medical word for the surgical removal of one breast, or both breasts. However, as it is with almost everything about breast cancer, there is no one surgical procedure you can point to and say, "That is, conclusively, what a mastectomy is." There are six different kinds of mastectomy and there is, additionally, a different procedure known as a lumpectomy that can be performed to remove breast tissue. All of the following surgical solutions to breast cancer are known as "local therapies", meaning that they target the cancer where it lives by excising it and a margin of surrounding healthy tissue; chemotherapy, on the other hand, is an example of a "systemic" solution.

- **Lumpectomy** (sometimes referred to as a partial mastectomy) involves the removal of breast tissue, but the amount of tissue removed is minimal and the breast is preserved. The procedure is a type of "wide local excision" (WLE), in which a small section of diseased tissue as well as a margin of healthy tissue is removed.

- **Simple mastectomy** (also called a 'total mastectomy') involves the removal of the entire breast, but axillary tissues such as lymph nodes are not removed, with the possible exception of the sentinel lymph node, or the first axillary lymph node. The lymph nodes are similar to pearls on a string; the first pearl is the one closest to the breast and, so, the first into which any cancer that is in the process of metastasizing would be expected to drain. This first pearl is the sentinel node. I note here that the practice of sentinel node biopsy has saved a lot of women from extensive axillary node dissection, something that used to be a huge contributor to lymphedema.

- **Skin-sparing mastectomy** involves the removal of the problematic breast tissue through a small incision made around the areola, which is the dark skin that surrounds the nipple. Sparing the breast skin opens up more reconstruction options. However, not all patients are candidates for skin-sparing mastectomy—for example, patients who are diagnosed with cancers that involve the skin, such as inflammatory cancer.

- **Nipple-sparing mastectomy** involves the removal of the breast tissue while preserving the nipple and areola and the entire breast skin or envelope. In the past, this procedure has been used exclusively for women whose mastectomies were being done prophylactically, or for women with benign breast conditions that involved mastectomy as part of the treatment. This was because there was concern that cancer cells would either not be fully removed from or develop in the ductal tissues that remained around the spared nipple. Techniques are now sophisticated enough to make a nipple-sparing mastectomy a viable option for a broader range of patients, but long term data is still needed before this will become standard care for patients. It is important to know that women whose breasts are ptotic, meaning very large, or whose nipple position is too low or facing downward may not be candidates for nipple-sparing mastectomies.

- **Modified radical mastectomy** involves the removal of the entire breast as well as the fatty tissue and lymph nodes (also called 'axillary contents') surrounding the breast.

● **Radical mastectomy** (also called a 'Halsted mastectomy') involves the removal of the entire breast and the fatty tissues and lymph nodes, as well as the pectoral muscles and other minor muscles behind the breast. This procedure is rarely done and almost never indicated.

● **Extended radical mastectomy** involves the removal of the entire breast and the fatty tissues and lymph nodes, the pectoral muscles and other minor muscles behind the breast, AND the internal mammary lymph node chain that is located within the chest wall.

Breast Reconstruction

I believe the best way to begin our discussion of breast reconstruction techniques is to address the questions my patients ask most frequently. This should help to allay some basic concerns, and to lay the groundwork for more knowledgeable consideration of all the options available to patients after a mastectomy.

First, immediate breast reconstruction does not interfere with chemotherapy and may not interfere with radiation treatments that follow surgery. According to a study by the National Institutes of Health, even though reconstruction may, in some cases, delay the initiation of chemo, it doesn't mean a patient will not be able to have chemo, or that the start of the prescribed chemotherapy treatment will be significantly delayed.[132] The question is: does it matter if immediate breast reconstruction delays the initiation of chemotherapy? The answer is NO.[133] Studies continue to show that women who have immediate breast reconstruction have similar survival rates and local recurrence rates to women who did not undergo immediate breast reconstruction.

The answer to whether reconstruction will get in the way of adjuvant therapy is a little more complicated if the therapy in question is radiation. That is because radiation can sometimes cause damage to a reconstructed breast, particularly if implants have been used. If a woman knows she will need radiation therapy after surgery, and that she will want or need to use implants as part of her reconstruction plan, her plastic surgeon might recommend that she delay reconstruction until after the radiation therapy course is complete. Sometimes, however, a woman does not know whether or not she will need to undergo radiation therapy until *after* her mastectomy, when she and her doctor have been able to assess the surgery event and/or her pathology report. As radiation therapy is being utilized for more and more patients and is necessary for almost all patients undergoing breast conservation or lumpectomy, it is important to understand how you will specifically benefit

---

132 *http://www.ncbi.nlm.nih.gov/pmc/articles/PMC3268930/.*

133 ³"Long-term clinical outcome of immediate reconstruction after mastectomy," R. Riefkohl Georgiade, E. Cox *et al.,* Plastic Reconstructive Surgery, 76: 415–420 (1985); "Oncological outcome after immediate breast reconstruction for invasive breast cancer: a long-term study," Breast,13: 210-218 (2004); "Patterns of local breast cancer recurrence after skin-sparing mastectomy and immediate breast reconstruction" The American Journal of Surgery, 194: 438-443 (2007).

from radiation, as demonstrated from clinical studies, because very little time is focused on the permanent negative effects of radiation. Unlike chemotherapy, where the effects wash out of your system with time in most instances, radiation therapy has permanent effects including decreased blood flow, possible injury to your heart and lungs, and significant fibrosis (tightening and scarring) of your chest wall. Now, in some patients, radiation can significantly decrease local recurrence after a mastectomy and therefore the benefits greatly outweigh the risks. So the primary message here is you should talk to your radiation oncologist to ensure that the recommended radiation treatment will be a true benefit to you. This is another reason why we refer to your doctors—particularly in this case your general surgeon, your radiation oncologist, and your plastic surgeon—as a team: if radiation is a possibility following mastectomy, all three doctors will need to have this information to be able to advise you most appropriately.

The next most frequently asked question, then, has to do with *when* the reconstruction surgery can be performed. The answer depends on the individual woman and her unique cancer experience, but the broad answer is that reconstruction surgery can take place immediately following mastectomy—that is, your plastic surgeon will follow your general surgeon into the operating room as soon as your mastectomy is complete, to begin the reconstruction process. Or it can also be delayed. As we've already discussed, it's sometimes beneficial to delay the reconstruction surgery when radiation therapy follows mastectomy. Another valid reason for delaying breast reconstruction can be that the patient simply isn't ready for it yet. Delaying the reconstruction surgery can allow you the time you might need to consider all your reconstruction options.

On the other hand, there is a lot to be said for the benefits of breast reconstruction in general, of course, and for immediate breast reconstruction (IBR) in particular: patients who experienced IBR have a pronounced psychological advantage during the healing process.[134] One of the reasons for this is the patient doesn't wake up from her surgery with a flat mastectomy scar on her chest. As Julie said to me when her reconstruction was complete, "I never had a day without my ta-tas! They were always there when I looked in the mirror at myself." Also, while the results can be very good with delayed reconstructions, your doctor will often be able to achieve better, more aesthetic results with immediate breast reconstruction.

Another question is about scarring and what the reconstructed breast will look like. This is so variable from woman to woman and breast to breast that it's hard to answer specifically. Some general surgeons can and will do a mastectomy through a circular incision. This is obviously a more challenging surgery, but, when reconstructed, the scar may disappear in the areola and nipple. Some incisions are horizontal across the breast, and these can prove challenging to cover with bathing suits, depending on how long the scar is and how revealing the bathing suit is. Scarring with a nipple sparing procedure produces yet another scar on the skin. Lumpectomy will obviously result in a

---

134 *http://www.ncbi.nlm.nih.gov/pubmed/6131178/.*

scar wherever the tumor is located. But the thing that surprised Julie is something we might not routinely discuss, and that is the scar tissue that forms at the chest wall when the breast is completely removed. Just like the scar tissue in the armpit that needs to be regularly worked and massaged and stretched, the scar tissue on the chest wall can contract down if it's not managed well post-operatively. It can cover a large area and be much more significant than the axillary scar tissue, depending on the individual woman and her individual procedure. Most patients will benefit from a post-operative guided physical therapy session, even if for just a few sessions, to learn the proper way to perform various exercises and massages.

Always among the top questions are ones about insurance coverage of reconstruction procedures. In 1999, the Women's Health and Cancer Rights Act (WHCRA) was passed. This law requires group health plans, HMOs and insurance companies that offer coverage for mastectomy to also cover reconstructive surgery after mastectomy. This coverage must also include, by law, reconstruction of the unaffected breast in order to achieve a more balanced look, breast prostheses, and the treatment of all physical complications that are associated with the mastectomy. That said, Medicare and Medicaid recipients are not covered by WHCRA, and some insurance plans sponsored through religious organizations may also be exempt from compliance with this law, so it is always advisable for a patient to speak with her insurance company prior to choosing her method of reconstruction in order to determine what is and is not covered by her individual policy.

Finally—sadly—I am also often asked why I insist my patients quit smoking before I perform their reconstruction surgery. I don't do it because I am violently opposed to smoking—which, like most doctors today, I am—but because it can cause real and significant post-surgery complications, including complications around wound healing due to decreased circulation of blood to the skin. These complications are seen immediately, not ten to twenty years in the future, as in the case of lung cancer. One cigarette decreases the capillary blood flow for two hours, thereby contributing to skin loss or delayed healing, which can ultimately result in having to remove the reconstructed breasts and start over. Therefore I ask all my patients who are undergoing breast reconstruction surgery to quit smoking prior to the surgery—and I extract a promise from them they will stay smoke-free after surgery as well.

Your Options for Breast Reconstruction after Mastectomy

Broadly speaking, there are three 'categories' of options available for breast reconstruction. In this section, I'll explain all three of these categories in some depth, the advantages and disadvantages of each, and particular characteristics of the different surgical techniques that may make one more, or less, appropriate for your individual reconstruction needs and desires.

The categories are:

- **Mastectomy only** with breast prosthesis

- **Implant-based** reconstruction

- **Reconstruction** using only your own tissue

Mastectomy Only with Breast Prosthesis

Treatments—and prognoses—for breast cancer have improved dramatically over the years, as have outcomes for reconstruction surgery. But that doesn't mean that everyone will need or want to take advantage of surgical reconstruction options. Some women may be entirely comfortable with a treatment process that involves removal of the breast, with or without axillary lymph node sampling as necessary, and then, when the incisions have healed, being fitted for a breast prosthesis. Prostheses are sometimes described as hot and uncomfortable, but the advantage of this minimal post-mastectomy course is that no further surgery is needed after breast removal. The entire mastectomy process usually takes no more than one to two hours, so the patient is under anesthesia for a very limited period of time, and she can be home and healing after just one day in the hospital.

WHAT HAPPENS IF A BREAST IMPLANT RUPTURES?

Saline

If a saline implant ruptures, the breast will change in shape and size as the implant deflates. Surgery is then required to remove the ruptured implant from the breast, but the saline fluid itself—salt water—is absorbed by the body with no risk to the woman's health. Rupture rate for saline implants used for reconstructive purposes is generally 1% per year.

Silicone

It's hard to tell if a silicone implant has ruptured as the silicone gel has a tendency to become trapped in the capsule of fibrous tissue that your body forms naturally around the implant. This does not mean that, eventually, a ruptured silicone implant will not cause breast pain, or changes in the size and shape of the breast, in which case surgery will be required to address the problem. There is currently no documented evidence that leaking silicone can itself be the cause of disease or other health problems. Rupture rate for silicone implants is similar to that for saline implants. For most patients, the implants will last ten to fifteen years.

Implant-based Reconstruction

Implant-based reconstruction places either a saline or a silicone implant under the pectoralis muscle to reconstruct the breast. Both saline and silicone implants have a similar outer shell, but there are subtle differences between the two types. Saline implants are filled with sterile salt water; they are empty when your plastic surgeon implants them in your body and filled only once they are in place. Silicone implants are pre-filled with a thick silicone gel that has a look and feel very similar to natural body fat. There are numerous shapes, profiles, and sizes of both saline and silicone gel implants—indeed, even as I was editing this chapter, two new styles of silicone gel implants have been approved by the FDA. So talk to your plastic surgeon about the advantages or disadvantages of the different types of implants to find one that best suits your desires and needs.

An important note: When you consider an implant-based reconstruction, you have to take into account the amount of skin that will be available after your mastectomy. It is advantageous, then, if your doctor is able to perform a skin-sparing mastectomy. Depending on the amount of skin, your desired cup size, and the health of the skin flaps created by the general surgeon, you may have either a one-stage direct-to-implant reconstruction or a two-stage tissue-expander reconstruction. Two-stage tissue-expander reconstruction is the most commonly employed method of reconstruction and has been able to produce reliable, aesthetically pleasing results with a

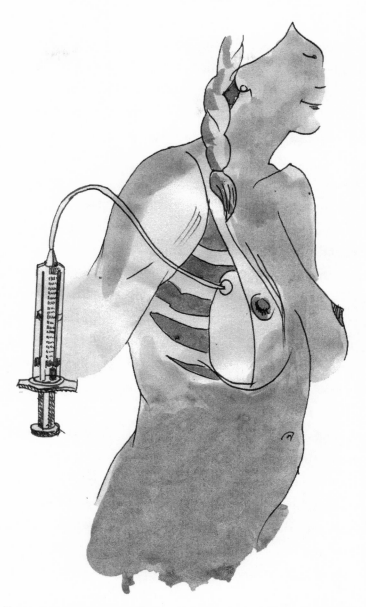

Two-stage tissue-expander reconstruction is the most commonly employed method of reconstruction. A tissue expander is placed under the pectoralis muscle and expanded over the next several months in your doctor's office.

low complication rate. A tissue expander is placed under the pectoralis muscle and expanded over the next several months, about every one to two weeks, in your doctor's office. When the expander is fully expanded, the final implant surgery takes place. If necessary, nipple/areola reconstruction then completes your reconstruction.

What are the advantages of choosing to have implant-based reconstruction? Well, the implant can provide fullness to the upper breast, giving a more youthful appearance to the breast, and the extra volume of the implant can help to correct ptosis, or loose, drooping skin, of the breast. Additionally, your recovery time from implant-based reconstruction is generally faster than with reconstruction methods that use only your own tissue, and there are no additional scars on the body at the tummy, buttock, or other donor site. Plus, you can get away with *not* wearing a bra, an added bonus that appeals to some of my patients.

But let's weigh those advantages against the disadvantages: an implant is an implant is an implant—there is no getting around the fact that it is a foreign object in the body. This means that there is the increased risk of infection around the implant, and the implant will one day rupture, statistically between ten to fifteen years after surgery. This will require another surgery, but removal and replacement of a ruptured implant is a relatively straightforward procedure that is performed in an outpatient setting. The shape of the breast may be less 'natural' with an implant and the capsule of tissue that the body may naturally form around the implant can become firm, and may become painful in a small percentage of patients. Further, using an expander requires two stages (surgeries) for complete reconstruction, and the expansion itself, done in semi-weekly visits to your doctor's office, can be uncomfortable and even painful.

Latissimus Muscle with Implant

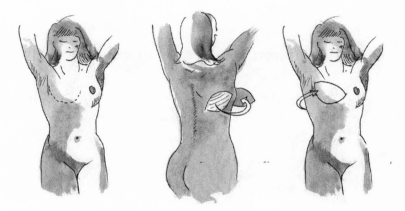

The lat flap method of reconstruction is most often used for either patients who are undergoing delayed reconstruction after radiation therapy and do not have enough tummy fat, or for patients who have had a prior lumpectomy with radiation and now, due to a number of different circumstances, require a salvage mastectomy.

This is a technique that is usually but not always combined with a breast implant. Since it is a procedure I perform with regularity, I want to describe it here.

The latissimus muscle, commonly known as the "lat", and the skin is removed from the patient's back and 'tunneled' to the front of the chest wall where it is formed into a new breast mound. This new mound is then combined, or enhanced, with the implant or a tissue expander. The advantages of this method of reconstruction include that the lat flap can bring unirradiated or unburnt tissue to the breast area to help mitigate the effects of the radiation treatment. More to the point, however, I use this technique for two subgroups of patients:

1. Patients who undergo delayed reconstruction after they have had radiation therapy and who do not have enough tummy fat or do not wish to use their tummy tissue.

2. Patients who have had a lumpectomy with radiation in the past and now, due to a number of different circumstances, require a salvage mastectomy.

There are enormous advantages to this method and other methods that use the patient's own tissue from a donor site. But they should be carefully weighed with the drawbacks, including the risk that fluid can collect back at that donor site, which it does in about 15% of patients after the drains have been removed.

Reconstruction Using Only Your Own Tissue

The alternative to implant-based breast reconstruction is *autologous breast reconstruction*. *Autologous* is a medical term for donor tissue that comes from the recipient rather than a donor; this method of breast reconstruction, then, involves using your body's own tissue to reconstruct your breast or breasts after mastectomy. When skin, fat, and sometimes muscle are harvested from one site on the body and transferred from the original site to another place on the body, the *composite* tissue—composite because it is composed of skin, fat and possibly muscle—is referred to as a *flap*. In the case of breast reconstruction, your plastic surgeon uses the flap to recreate and shape the breast mound.

There are several natural advantages in opting for autologous reconstruction—you are using your own tissue so, unlike implants, it will never spring a leak or need to be replaced. Additionally, using your own tissues creates a very natural appearing breast that will change with you as you gain or lose weight and that will never rupture. A successful autologous reconstruction will last for a lifetime. However—you were expecting this, of course—there are disadvantages. The immediate concern is that reconstructions that involve your own tissue are more complex and involved procedures than those that are implant-based, so you can expect surgery to be significantly longer, depending on the particular procedure you choose and other circumstances unique to your cancer experience. The amount of time under anesthesia is reduced when the reconstructive surgeon is a reconstructive team. I usually do autologous reconstructions with my partner if we're doing two sides, so that there is less anesthesia time for our patients. In addition, there is a donor site to consider, meaning a scar to heal and recover from somewhere else, although in most cases where the tummy tissue is used, women are not sad to see their belly fat gone.

Methods of "flap" reconstruction include the TRAM, SIEA, DIEP, SGAP, IGAP, and TUG—acronyms that refer primarily to the location of the donor site (whether the flap comes from the tummy or the gluteals, for example), though there are other distinctions among the methods that are substantial. Let's discuss each of these methods in more detail:

- **Pedicled TRAM,** Transverse Rectus Abdominal Myocutaneous, or pTRAM

- **Free TRAM,** Transverse Rectus Abdominal Myocutaneous, or fTRAM

- **Muscle-sparing TRAM,** Transverse Rectus Abdominal Myocutaneous

- **SIEA,** Superficial Inferior Epigastric Artery

- **DIEP,** Deep Inferior Epigastric Perforator

- **SGAP,** Superior Gluteal Artery Perforator

- **IGAP,** Inferior Gluteal Artery Perforator

- **TUG,** Transvere Upper Gracilis

Pedicled TRAM

Medical terms, when you get down to root definitions, are usually pretty straightforward. In this case, when you know that,
in biology, the word pedicle means a small, stalk-like structure
connecting one organ to another, you can more easily visualize how this method of breast reconstruction works: the skin,

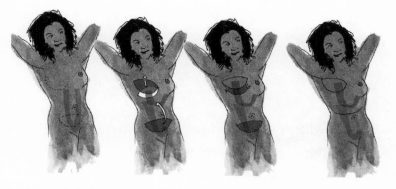

In the pedicled TRAM method of breast reconstruction, the skin,
fat, and a portion of the abdominal muscle is transferred to the
chest area by rotating it and tunneling it under your skin.

fat, and a portion of the rectus abdominus muscle—that is,
what you refer to at the gym as your *abs*—is transferred as
one composite unit, or flap, to the chest area to recreate your
breast by rotating it and tunneling it under your skin. Tunneling the flap makes it unnecessary to separate the blood vessels
that supply that flap of tissue from the body. The risks that
follow this surgery include the significant potential for hernia due to the removal of a portion of the abdominal muscle,

and for *fat necrosis*, or areas that feel more firm, to develop in the migrated tissue. In addition, since the rectus abdominus muscle is removed, women lose their core strength and some have difficulty getting up from bed or a chair. Due to the inherent risks associated with a pedicle TRAM, and since there are other less invasive ways to achieve the same result, I would NOT recommend a pedicled TRAM procedure for any of my patients. If your plastic surgeon recommends a pedicled TRAM, you may want to ask about other options that have fewer complications.

Free TRAM

This procedure uses the same flap of tissue as the Pedicled TRAM except only the lower portion of the rectus abdominus muscle is removed. In addition, in this case the abdominal tissue is disconnected before the flap is transferred to the breast pocket. The blood supply is then reconnected under a microscope to a new source under the arm or chest. The benefits of an fTRAM over a pTRAM are that a smaller portion of the abdominals is usually involved so the risk of hernia is decreased; at the same time, the supply of blood to the donor tissue is usually increased.

Muscle-sparing TRAM

With the procedure known as the muscle-sparing TRAM, the flap that is used is the same except that even less muscle, often only a small strip, is removed and left attached to the flap. As with the fRAM, the blood supply is disconnected before the

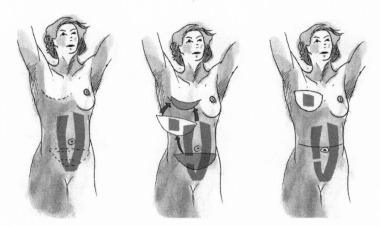

The free TRAM method of reconstruction is similar to the pedicled TRAM method, except only the lower portion of the abdominal muscle is removed, and it is disconnected before the flap is transferred to the breast pocket. The blood supply is then reconnected under a microscope to a new source under the arm or the chest.

tissue is relocated to the chest area and then reconnected under a microscope to a new supply under the arm or chest. The advantage here is clear: while you will still have to be protective of your tummy while it heals at the donor site, less of your core muscles—and strength—are disturbed.

If you opt to undergo a TRAM procedure, you can expect to be in the hospital for three to five days, with an overall recovery time of four to six weeks, and your doctor will likely advise you not to lift anything weighing more than ten pounds for at least six weeks. Advantages of opting for a TRAM procedure? It can give an excellent aesthetic result, especially for women with larger breasts with moderate ptosis, with the additional aesthetic appearance of a tummy tuck. The disadvantages? About 5% of patients will experience an abdominal hernia, and about 1-2% of cases require a re-operative procedure to correct an inadequate supply of blood to the flap, or even the loss of the flap. There is also a slightly increased risk for DVT (deep vein thrombosis) or blood clots in the leg, and of blood loss and, therefore, the need for transfusion.

This brings up the question of blood transfusion. Although it's rarely needed for these procedures, you should discuss the possibility with your surgical team. Depending on the timing of your surgery with your other breast cancer treatment, you might be able to donate blood ahead of time for your own use if it's needed. Julie felt very strongly about not having transfusion if it was at all possible. There are ways to keep the body stable without using blood most of the time. We agreed that there would only be transfusion if she was what we call "hemodynamically unstable," meaning that she didn't have enough blood cells to keep her vital life processes going without adding blood to her circulatory system.

Perforator Flap Breast Reconstruction

One of the newer advances in autologous breast reconstruction is the development of *perforator flaps*. Using the perforator flap method allows for an even more elegant type of reconstruction in which no muscle is taken, only the fat and skin necessary to recreate a breast. The blood vessels necessary to keep the flap alive are microsurgically dissected *through* the muscle, and then they are reconnected to a new blood supply in the chest or under the arm. Because the blood supply is so critical to these types of surgery, you may be asked to have a special CT scan to evaluate your blood vessels prior to your reconstruction. By sparing the muscle altogether, patients have less pain at the donor site, faster recovery time, and lower hernia rate. Microsurgical breast reconstruction has a high rate of success—98%—and provides soft, pliable skin and fat that help to create a natural-looking and aesthetically pleasing breast. Unlike some of the implant surgery, a bra has to be worn in order to support the new breast.

There are four primary types of perforator flap methods:

- **DIEP Flap**
  - Patients who have a moderate amount of abdominal wall skin and fat are excellent candidates for DIEP

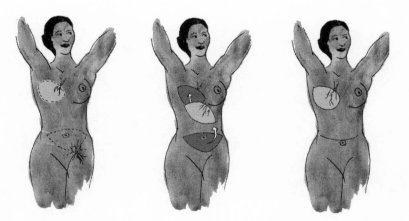

In DIEP Flap reconstruction skin and fat are detached from the lower abdomen and relocated to the chest to form the new breast.

385

Flap breast reconstruction. The skin and fat are detached from the lower abdomen and relocated to the chest where they are artistically molded to recreate a natural-looking breast. Microsurgery is used to hook up the arteries and veins to new sources and restore the blood flow to the tissue.

● SIEA Flap
 • This method is very similar to a DIEP Flap, except that when the tummy skin and fat and necessary blood vessels are removed for transfer to the chest wall, the abdominal wall *fascia* is left untouched along with the abdominal muscles. Fascia is the band or layer of fibrous connective tissue that surrounds our muscles. By leaving the fascia intact, the SIEA Flap is even less invasive than the DIEP flap, and the risk of hernia is eliminated since there are no fascial incisions. Further, the bonus tummy tuck yields improved, or flatter, results. The downside of the SIEA Flap alternative is that only a small percentage of patients— about 5%—are candidates for the procedure. The issue is that the superficial blood vessels that are used to supply blood to the flap after it has been relocated are very small, and that limits the size of the flap as well as increases the risk of its loss. Patients who have had prior abdominal surgery, such as Caesarian section or a hysterectomy, are generally not good candidates for a SIEA Flap.

- ### SGAP Flap and IGAP Flap

  - These flap procedures involve the buttocks as donor tissue sites and can be an alternative for women who have very little abdominal tissue, or who have had prior surgeries that will eliminate the DIEP Flap or TRAM Flap as options. But for a variety of reasons, these procedures are not routinely recommended. The skin of the buttocks is less pliable and soft, and shaping the new breast is more difficult, for one thing. The complexity of reattaching the small blood vessels located in the buttock area of the body means that these procedures take more time than the DIEP or SIEP Flap options. Finally, the buttock that is the donor site will have some change in contour, creating asymmetry, though this can be successfully covered with clothing. On the plus side: the gluteal muscle is spared, and since the abdominal muscles are not touched, patients generally have a faster recovery time.

- ### TUG flap

  - This procedure involves using tissue from the inner thigh. As with SGAP and IGAP procedures, the abdominal muscles are not touched so recovery time is usually faster. However, TUG flap reconstruction is in the main reserved for women who don't have a lot of abdominal tissue, possibly because they've had a tummy tuck in the past, or who want smaller breasts because there is generally not a lot of excess fat distri-

387

bution in this area of the body. It is appropriate to call the SGAP, IGAP, and TUG flap procedures "backup options"—if you look at all the flap procedures done, all the procedures performed that use the patient's own tissue, 95% of them use abdominal tissue and a mere 5% use either gluteal or thigh tissue.

How do a patient and her doctor make a decision about where donor tissue will be taken? There will be a few unique-to-the-patient reasons in every case, but, in general, much of the decision will be based on how much tissue is available at the chosen site for her surgeon to harvest.

Nipple Reconstruction

Nipple reconstruction is usually the final milestone in your complete breast-reconstruction journey. There are many techniques to accomplish it, and there isn't one of them that's going to be wholly satisfactory for every woman. Some women, unwilling to have another surgery, are going to be happy with their new breasts and opt out of nipple reconstruction altogether. Julie, for instance, thought that she was satisfied without doing the nipple reconstruction. But I have always felt that there is a real aesthetic value to the nipple reconstruction as our eye is accustomed to seeing a nipple on a breast. The color variations that nipple reconstruction creates unconsciously draw one's attention away from the scars, and most women have a feeling of wholeness after they undergo nipple-areola

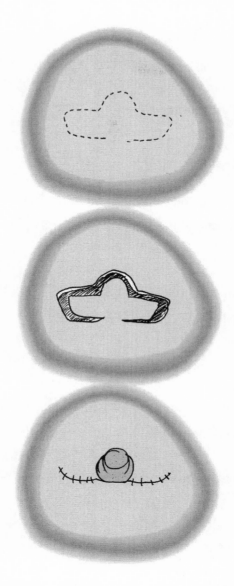

If you desire to have the nipple project or stick out a little, your plastic surgeon will often perform a minor surgical procedure to bring together small skin flaps from the breast itself to create a projecting mound of tissue. The areola reconstruction can then be performed via secondary tattoo or a skin graft.

reconstruction. After we did her nipple reconstruction, Julie agreed that it made a real visual difference.

There are a number of options for nipple-areola reconstruction. If you desire to have the nipple project or stick out a little, your plastic surgeon will often perform a minor surgical procedure to bring together small skin flaps from the breast itself to create a projecting mound of tissue. The areola reconstruction can then be performed via secondary tattoo or a skin graft. Others are going to be delighted with the non-surgical option of undergoing 3D nipple reconstruction in which one tattoos the areola and a three- dimensional, shaded nipple is created—although if you are considering this option, you will want to ask your plastic surgeon about the quality of the ink she or he uses; many tattoo inks get their "permanence" due to heavy metals such as lead or mercury in their formulas.[135] Julie's daughter was actually the family member who asked about tattoo ink when her family came in to discuss the planned surgery, and I was glad to be able to tell her that the medical grade tattoo ink we use did not contain any heavy metals.

For most patients undergoing implant-based reconstruction, there is very little to no light-touch sensation in most of the breast or the newly reconstructed nipple. This is similar for even nipple-sparing mastectomy patients since the nerves coming through the breast tissue that is removed are cut. Patients undergoing autologous breast reconstruction can have some

---

135 *http://www.scientificamerican.com/article.cfm?id=tattoo-ink-mercury-and-other-toxins.*

return of sensation with time (usually one year) since the nerves can regrow through their own tissue; however, sensation is never what it once was.

A NOTE FROM JULIE ABOUT BREAST AND NIPPLE SENSATIONS

During my surgery, Ankit did perform nerve relocation for me, the goal of which is to help with the sensory recovery piece. Not all surgeons can or will do this, and if yours does you will want to be aware that even with nerve relocation it will still take what seems like forever—up to a year—to feel anything, as nerves grow very slowly.

One thing I wish I had known as I came out of surgery was how much the changes in sensation would affect the way I hugged. I couldn't feel the people I was hugging anymore, and I didn't know how hard to squeeze, and so I didn't feel as if I'd really had a hug. This improved within a few months, as sensation returned, but even having taken advantage of the nerve-relocation option that was available to me, I still miss the sensations I used to feel in my nipples. I don't miss them standing up when I'm cold at all, but I do miss them in intimate settings.

Recovering After Breast Reconstruction

Generally, patients remain in the hospital for one to seven days after breast reconstruction surgery, the length of time being dependent on the type of reconstruction that has been performed. As Julie mentioned in the previous chapter, most reconstructive surgeries of the breast require the use of post-operative drains. Drains are simply tubes that are used to allow blood, pus, or other fluids to drain from the surgical wound. The drains are routinely needed for only a short period of time, often one week. During this time, your doctor will likely ask you to wear special post-surgical garments or binders as well; these are compression garments that support your new breast or breasts, your tummy or other donor site, and help to reduce swelling and bruising. If your reconstruction has involved a flap method, you will be monitored closely every hour in the first days, to make sure there is adequate blood flow to the flap. Additionally, your doctor will likely prescribe blood thinners for a day or two, to prevent the possibility of blood clots.

As with many surgeries, you will likely be encouraged to ambulate—that is, to get up and start walking—quite quickly after your surgery. The post-operative period is a time for rest—and a time when most patients are more than inclined to do so—so why do we ask you to get up and pace the hallways as soon after surgery as possible? For a lot of great reasons! When you walk, however slowly, you are using the large muscles in your legs, and that gets your blood flowing through your body, which, in turn, speeds the healing process of your wounds. Walking also helps get your urinary tract and gastro-intestinal functions—functions that slow down when you're under anesthesia and receiving pain medication—back up to speed, and it decreases the risk of everything from blood clots to constipation and gas pains. So, after surgery, start walking slowly or with assistance—because you may feel weak or dizzy and you don't want to push yourself too hard at first—but do *start* because it is one of the most positive, proactive things you can do to restore your health. And you can begin to do it while you're still in the hospital!

10

Exercise!

If you exercise because you want a smaller butt
or because you want to fit into a smaller dress,
you may or may not exercise until you reach those
small goals. Instead, exercise because it feels
good, because it makes you happy, because
you love how your skin glows after you do it.
Exercise because you are saving your own life.

Julie

Some people—too many people, I
fear—think of exercise as an optional activity. I can't tell you
the times I have *beseeched* patients to add some physical
activity to their daily, or even weekly, routines.

I always have a great chuckle at the TV ads for cholesterol
meds that say "When diet and exercise fail..." The truth is
that diet and exercise don't fail. *We fail to do them.* So when
I'm told—*diet and exercise don't work*, I have many replies. No,
they don't; not if we do them for only a day, or a week, or even
a month though, by the end of one month we may achieve
some temporary goal like fitting into a smaller-sized dress in
time for our college reunion or last year's bathing suit in time
for this year's swim season. We may feel good if we meet our
short-term goal, but if we haven't incorporated activity into our
lifestyle, rather than merely used it as a means to look better at
a special event, we aren't going to sustain the new, improved
look—and we aren't going to sustain the health benefits we've
achieved during the time when we were active.

Remember how in Chapter One we talked about the body
as a symphonic machine? How the health of every part of it is

critical to the health of the whole in the same way a timpani and a piccolo are both critical if an orchestra wants to perform Beethoven's Fifth? Well, now I want you to take that metaphor one step further—I want you to think about how beautiful a piece of music is when all of the separate instruments playing it are in good working order and well-tuned. And then I want you to think about how painful the performance could be on your ear if the piccolo was rusty, the violin was missing its E string, and the tension on the timpani's heads hadn't been equalized. Exercise fine tunes all your separate parts and keeps them in good working order so you can perform your *life* beautifully—it gets the blood flowing to keep your veins and arteries clean and open, it keeps your joints juicy and flexible, it keeps your bones and muscles sleek and strong, it helps keep the conversation going among all the cells in your brain so you can think clearly.

If you already exercise regularly, then read this chapter to find out why exercise is even more critical to you as a cancer survivor, and what exercises can offer even greater benefits to your sustained, post-cancer health. If you view exercise as something odious that you do only under duress, only when you want to drop a few pounds or are guilted into it by a doctor or a friend or your partner, I beseech you to allow me to help you change the scenery—I'm asking you to read this chapter as if your life depended on it.

Because it does.

Now, I'm not suggesting that you become a long distance runner, or that you get a gym membership and a personal trainer and start pumping iron. Most of us aren't Olympic-caliber athletes and we don't have to become one in order to incorporate adequate exercise into our lives. We just have to do the right kinds of exercises regularly, consistently, and mindfully. The benefits of mild, and even minimal exercise—often the only kind that busy women have time for—can do wonders as we regain, and then sustain, our health. A common sense approach is what we want to achieve.

What can regular exercise do for you?

Heart disease, diabetes and cancer are among the top ten diseases in America.[136] One of the primary risk factors for heart disease is a sedentary lifestyle; moderate exercise—just thirty minutes a day—can lower blood pressure, reduce "bad" cholesterol and increase "good" cholesterol, and so help to prevent what is, as of this writing, the nation's number one killer. Regular exercise helps the body to use insulin to control glucose (sugar) levels—information that diabetics, and those who don't want to become diabetics, should take to heart. I'm about to tell you all about how exercise can help to prevent cancer, to be part of its cure, and to make sure that it doesn't recur. Let's start with the three categories of exercise you need to be doing on a regular basis: cardio or endurance, strength training or weight training, and stretching.

---

136 *http://www.cdc.gov/nchs/fastats/lcod.htm.*

Cardio/Endurance

Some people think of the breast cancer walks that have become ubiquitous around the country as a way of raising funds for breast cancer research. They are that—and in this purpose do just a whole heap of good—but there is larger poetry about them as well: they are *walks*; they are big, showy, happy demonstrations of what we all, as cancer survivors, should be doing every day—or, at least five days a week. Ankit even has a regular walking group made up of former patients, so important does he consider this form of exercise.

Walking is one of the best ways we can take our cardiovascular exercise. Of course, if you enjoy running, or swimming, or some other form of cardio, by all means, continue to do what you like. The key to maintaining a cardio routine, as with any part of your exercise routine, is to choose an activity that you like. If you like something, you will continue to do it; just some of that common sense we were talking about!

If, however, you're just starting out on a regular cardio routine, let me recommend walking to you. Why? First, it is easy on the body—running is an example of a high impact form of cardio, which means it can be tough on the joints, but walking is low impact. Second, it is essentially cost free—you walk out your front door and get going. Third, you can do it anywhere, without any special equipment other than a pair of good, sturdy shoes; I travel a great deal, to speak at conferences and to see far-flung patients, and wherever I am going in the world all I have to remember to pack to keep up my cardio routine is my walking shoes.

I began my walking routine right after I was diagnosed, so I must say that, of course, I was gentle with myself about how consistently I did my cardio while I was in the chemo phase of my treatment (which I underwent prior to surgery). Additionally, though I wanted to go back to walking shorter distances more slowly as soon as I could after surgery, I found walking even on the pleasant, paved sidewalks of my suburban neighborhood to be difficult—and through that difficulty discovered the elliptical trainer. Elliptical trainers, also called cross trainers, simulate a cross between walking or running and stair climbing, and can be set to the intensity level most appropriate to where you are in regaining your fitness after your treatments. If you can afford a membership at a gym where an elliptical is among the equipment, or to purchase an elliptical for your home, I highly recommend it as an alternative to walking—a gentle alternative when you are first getting back on your feet, and an on-going alternative when it rains!

In addition to the myriad well-known benefits of cardio-vascular exercise, there is one benefit that is particular to us as breast cancer survivors. This specific benefit is that cardio workouts help us to maintain an appropriate weight for our heights and frames. Why is maintaining an appropriate weight important for us? As we have discussed in various other places in this book, breast cancer can often be responsive to hormones, such as estrogen—and estrogen is stored in fat. The less fat we carry on our bodies, then, the less opportunity for a hormone-responsive cancer to recur.

How much cardio do we need? In my functional medicine world, we tell folks that they need 150 minutes of moderate exercise each week. We tell cancer survivors that they need 300 of those minutes each week. And we're very specific about what moderate exercise is: moderate exercise is vigorous enough to keep your heart rate sustained at 50 to 70% of its maximum. You can calculate your maximum heart rate by subtracting your age from 220. Now, if you like vigorous exercise, where your sustained heart rate is between 70 and 85% of maximum, then you only need 75 minutes per week, or 150 minutes if you're a cancer survivor. For those of you who don't like that much math in your exercise equation, there are other ways to define this moderate exercise goal. The first way is to walk for thirty minutes every day, at least five days a week, at a pace that allows you to cover at least one mile in that time frame. The second way is to work up to taking a minimum of 10,000 steps per day. Most people take 5,000 steps or less a day, but it isn't hard to increase the number of steps we take if we practice becoming aware of how easy it is to avoid taking them: escalators, elevators, and the drive-through lane at the bank are all modern conveniences that aren't necessarily convenient when it comes to our health. Try purchasing an inexpensive step counter you can clip to your waistband and taking the stairs instead of the elevator, or parking the car and strolling down the street to do your banking at an inside teller window.

Strength Training

Cardio will help melt fat, but strength training will help tone muscle—and toned muscles are *functional* muscles.

If you're just beginning a strength training program, remember to start with light weights—one or two pounds at most, and then gradually increase the weight you're working with as your muscles grow accustomed to the work. You can use hand weights, resistance bands, or, for many exercises such as squats, your own body weight. Here's a tip: your local sporting goods store will probably carry an assortment of weight-training equipment options, including weighted gloves and adjustable ankle weights. And if money is tight, remember that you can put a pound of rice in a baggie and use one of those in each hand.

How often to strength train? Aim for a minimum of two thirty-minute sessions a week with your weights, but remember not to work the same set of muscles two days in a row, except for your abdominals which you can work every day. I like to shoot for two days a week working my arms, and two days for my legs.

To get the most out of weight-training exercises, and to prevent injury while doing them, it helps to do them *mindfully*. You don't want to jerk the weight or lock your joints while you're working out as these are both ways of causing injury; you do want to remember to breathe naturally while you're doing your sets. I like to think about the muscle I am working with any particular exercise—this helps to isolate the muscle and intensify the exercise. It's also very important to move the body part you are exercising through its full range of motion so that you don't get short muscles that injure more easily. If you are doing a bicep curl, be sure to straighten your arm fully, without locking the joint, and curl it completely. Start with a low weight with which you can perform at least one set of eight repetitions, and try to work up to three sets of fifteen repetitions of each exercise, increasing the weight as you progress.

But which exercises should you do? You'll find some books Ankit and I recommend to help you put together a good program in the Resources section of this book. If it's affordable, a few sessions with a weight trainer is a good investment when you're just starting out. Often your local gym or YMCA has a pro who can provide this service at a reasonable price.

Stretching

In Chapter Eight we talked about how important stretching is as part of your preparation for mastectomy. In order to retain, and even increase your range of motion, as well as your overall flexibility and freedom of movement, it should continue to be a part of your post-cancer exercise routine. There are many good guides to stretching properly and safely—you will find the ones we like best in the Resources section of this book—

but let me advocate for my favorite form, yoga—but not just any yoga.

There are many different ways to practice yoga, different styles and teachers. Indeed, in some classes yoga practice can be cardio, strength training and stretching all rolled into one! What all yoga practices have in common is their focus on the breath and the flexibility the poses promote. What you want, however, is a practice that focuses additionally on the smooth flow from one pose to another, and on relaxation techniques. If you are not used to doing yoga, a good way to start is to find a beginner's class in a style known as *Hatha* yoga. Hatha yoga was developed in the Fifteenth Century as a way to physically prepare the body for meditation and a more physically demanding yoga practice. When practiced as intended, then, the movements in Hatha yoga challenge the body but do not overly stress it, and the breathing and meditation elements are calming and stress-relieving.

That said, the word "yoga" has come to reference, in our Western culture, a form of more or less rigorous physical exercise, with the meditation or relaxation component taking an often-distant second place, and the practice of various forms is really dependent on the teacher who is leading the class. Look around for a class and a teacher you like—whose class you can leave feeling both physically and emotionally refreshed. And *that* said, what you will find in almost any yoga class you attend is deep respect for individual abilities. Every good yoga teacher will periodically remind the members of his class to work at their own pace, or to modify poses that are too difficult. I have attended advanced yoga classes, because that was the only class that would fit that week in my schedule and, when the poses or the pace of the class went beyond my skill level, I felt perfectly at home dropping into Child's Pose for a rest. Yoga as I have come to love it focuses on the breath, is not a competitive experience, and should never hurt.

Exercise and Depression

There is one more huge benefit of exercise and that is the impact activity can have not only on what we think of as our 'physical' health, but on what we often call our 'mental' health. Within this context of discussing physical exercise, you will begin to see that it really isn't a separate thing from mental health. Our moods and emotions—how happy or sad or serene or anxious or angry or content we feel—are a product of the biochemical soup in our brains.

Breast cancer triggers all sorts of emotions, most of them negative—anger, sadness, resentment, fear. These emotions were certainly a part of my mental landscape after my diagnosis and, with a serious disease like cancer rocking my world, even at the time in which I was really rocking and reeling, I understood them to be perfectly reasonable and rather appropriate emotions to experience. While I recognized the validity of my emotions, however, I also knew I didn't want to feel that way. No one *wants* to feel miserable or scared! Moreover, there are ways to prevent these emotions—quite normal given the circumstances—from escalating into full-blown, clinical depression characterized by a prolonged period of hopelessness and despair. The folks at the National Cancer Institute at the National Institutes of Health have debunked a few myths about those of us who have battled cancer beautifully, simply by acknowledging them as myths:[137]

● **All people with cancer** are NOT depressed.

● **Depression** in a person with cancer is NOT normal.

● **Treatments** ARE helpful.

I recommend exercise as the first and possibly the most helpful step in dealing with the expected emotional lows of cancer, and in dealing depression a knock-out blow before it can ever take hold. Why? Because, among other positive changes it makes on our bodies as well as our brains, exercise can change the brain's biochemistry. It can, for example, increase your level of serotonin. Serotonin is a neurotransmitter—that is, a chemical naturally produced in your body that helps your brain cells talk to each other. And what does serotonin do for us? It helps to control our growth, our repro-

---

137 *http://www.cancer.gov/cancertopics/pdq/supportivecare/depression/ HealthProfessional/page1.*

ductive functions, and our moods. Whether we are in a good mood or a bad one is, in part, determined by the level of serotonin in our systems; even moderate exercise can elevate that level.

Researchers have also found that, after exercise, subjects had elevated levels of other biochemicals in their bloodstreams, specifically biochemical opioids[138] and endocannabinoids[139]—biochemicals that resemble morphine and cannabis—and these, in turn and indirectly, activate the body's production of dopamine,[140] yet another neurotransmitter that helps to regulate mood. Indeed, studies have been completed that demonstrate the same result among depressed patients who have been given antidepressants and patients who have been guided through a consistent exercise program.[141]

It is critically important for your physical health that you get a good hold on your mental health—this is true at any time, but especially while you are battling cancer. If the tools we are suggesting here don't help you to be able to find some joy and happiness in life, be sure to seek additional help. Speak to your doctor and make sure you get involved with a good support group or professional counseling.

---

138 http://cercor.oxfordjournals.org/content/18/11/2523.

139 http://www.harford.de/arne/articles/NeuroReport.pdf.

140 http://www.psychologytoday.com/blog/the-compass-pleasure/201104/exercise-pleasure-and-the-brain.

141 http://www.apa.org/monitor/2011/12/exercise.aspx.

Let's summarize. Exercise helps prevent cancer, helps us through cancer, and helps keep cancer from recurring. It makes us look better, and feel better—by fighting the depression that is unfortunately common in cancer patients. It reduces stress, increases flexibility, strengthens bones and keeps muscles supple. If we do it right, it isn't time-consuming or painful, and, depending on the type of exercise we choose, it costs almost nothing.

Have I convinced you to get out your walking shoes yet?

11

Hormones

Painting a Masterpiece After Breast Cancer Muddles the Colors

I love the painter Claude Monet. Just looking at one of his gardens I begin to feel tranquil, to physically experience stress leaving my body. One of my favorites of his paintings is Le Bassin Aux Nymphéas. I look at it in wonder—it isn't a "pink" painting, it's a green painting, a blue painting, but look closer and of course you have to wonder how he might have managed to paint such a masterpiece without any pink on his palette.

Julie

Hormones.

This is the most delicate of subjects, requiring the most delicate of balance in practice, and in how we talk about it. So far, in this book, we have talked about hormones here and there, as it's been required—in Chapter Seven, for example, when we talked about HER2 testing, or in Chapter Ten when we talked about the importance of exercise in maintaining a healthy weight because the hormone estrogen can influence the growth of certain types of cancer and estrogen is stored in fat. Two out of three women who are diagnosed with breast cancer will have the type that is influenced by estrogen, and in that situation, our hormones—the delicate balance of them that can maintain our physical health (think of their role in preventing osteoporosis), our emotional happiness (think of their role in preventing mood swings), and what we perceive as our femininity and even desirability (think of their role in preserving our libido)—suddenly are no longer our friends. We may perceive them as wreaking havoc and mayhem—believe they are no longer something we'll be able to trust to balance the same way through menopause and thereafter. Truthfully, they are not, or should not be among those things we grant primary importance when we are first diagnosed.

That's a bold and broad statement, so let me explain quickly what I mean by it. A full 95% of new cases of breast cancer will be diagnosed among women who are forty years or older.[142] I, myself, was in my mid-40s when I was diagnosed. What this means is that the majority of us will begin our breast cancer journeys in the perimenopause[143] stage of our lives or later. That we will find out we have breast cancer at a time in our lives when our natural child-bearing years are coming to an end and we will have, during the normal course of our lives, already either had our children, made our decision not to have them, or reconciled ourselves to the fact that we have been unable to become a biological parent. Therefore the challenge of preserving our fertility so we may preserve the option of having biological children after our breast cancer journey is never even on the table for the vast majority of us. And that is a blessing. There are so many different aspects of breast cancer that each patient will have to navigate on her own terms, based on her own preferences and her own unique manifestation of the disease, that my sympathy for those 3% who walk this path with the added burden of post-cancer fertility issues is enormous. Indeed, when I think about this 3% in terms of how cen-

---

142 http://www.cancer.org/acs/groups/content/@epidemiologysurveilance/documents/document/acspc-030975.pdf.

143 The time period in a woman's life during which she begins to make the natural transition to menopause, or permanent infertility.

tral being a mother is to my own life—the ways in which being a mother defines me and the way I live and love—the injustice of a young woman with breast cancer can provoke rage. Young women should not get breast cancer; we humans should not have made a world in which young women are exposed to the kinds of environmental and cultural stresses that cause their DNA to unravel and disease to take hold of their young bodies.

That said, I'm not lacking in sympathy for my peers, or women who are even older than I was when they are diagnosed. I dealt with my own diagnosis in ways that were, for the most part, utterly practical. But I admit to tremendous closet turmoil about this aspect of my cancer journey: I was terrified that after cancer I would no longer be a real woman. I worried that I was going to sprout a ton of facial hair. I was frightened I would become a dried up old prune instead of remaining a vibrant life force who would be able to continue to do the work I love, and do it at the crisp pace that energizes me. I feared that I would no longer be emotionally accessible when, due to cancer treatments, my hormonal balance was upended; I feared, because of my estrogen positive status, I would not have the tools I wanted available to me to cope with the impending chemotherapy-induced menopause I was facing.

As it turned out, none of those worries was valid. Why? Well, for one thing, during my cancer treatment, when I was tossed headlong into chemical menopause, I didn't even really notice the whole menopausal hullabaloo my body must have been enduring. And that is because—shocking as this may be to admit—chemotherapy is such a miserable experience you really can't be bothered to notice a hot flash or yet another mood swing. It is only after cancer treatments are over that in the vast majority of cases one will, or, as I've indicated *should*, become concerned about the hormones that may or may not be present and/or balanced in the body. After treatment was over, I had to take stock, make sure that I was not making "pro-estrogenic" choices and, yet, give myself a little leeway for living and loving my life. Handling hormones in breast cancer is not a short-term, but a long-term consideration.

Let's begin our discussion of this long-term consideration by asking what may seem like a totally unrelated question: How does a painter know when a painting is done? When she has used just the right amount of color in just the right place on the canvas? That she has not been too heavy-handed with the blue or too ungenerous with the yellow? Too little of one color may make the painting feel unfinished. Too much of too many colors will turn the canvas to mud. Yet, when no color is hazarded, there is no painting at all. This is very much akin to the dilemma nearly every woman in the world will face when she enters the perimenopausal and then the menopausal stages of her life; this dilemma is no different for breast cancer patients, though the stakes of the solution she chooses may well be higher.

But let's look at the solutions we're able to choose as, in their way, luxuries. The generation of women who are now at greatest risk of developing breast cancer—the Baby Boom generation—are living lives that are longer, and likely much more active than any generation that has come before them. When their mothers reached menopause, either the natural or the chemically-induced sort we usually experience with chemotherapy, they didn't have the luxury of the advanced reconstruction options our generation enjoys, to say nothing of the option to replace or replenish their hormones. They had their mastectomies, bought their prothesetic bras, and got on with it. Obsession with retaining our youth—of not putting away the things of youth and growing gracefully into a new age—is a relatively recent phenomenon, and one that is more of a social construct than a natural one. I'm in no way implying that we shouldn't take advantage of the ways we can now take to retain our vigor; I am advocating for a thoughtful approach to what living as a post-menopausal breast cancer survivor might mean.

For example, after my chemo was over and my breast surgery was complete, I was offered the option of taking estrogen-blocking drugs. This offer came because I had not had a hysterectomy as part of my treatment; I still had my ovaries and they would continue to manufacture estrogen and, left to their own devices, they might produce enough estrogen to trigger a recurrence of cancer. The estrogen-blocking drugs would make it so I wouldn't have to worry about what my ovaries were trying to do.

I had a lot of girlfriends—medical professionals, functional medicine buddies—who were rooting for me during my cancer experience, and one of the things they were rooting for was that I keep my ovaries and stay the course with an as natural and normal-as-possible approach. This is a viable and realistic and doable approach, one that many, many women choose.

But I was freaked out by my ovaries. The idea that they were manufacturing and releasing estrogen all through my body was a nightmare for me. I had no peace. Until one day it suddenly occurred to me that the stress of trying to keep my ovaries was causing me a bigger problem than the ovaries themselves. I realized that I was considering whether or not to keep my ovaries based on what my medical family, my peers and mentors and friends, ideally, believed in medically. So I had a conversation with my husband. His reaction? *What was I waiting for? Go, have a hysterectomy. Do whatever I needed to do to find peace, and to make sure that we never had to go through cancer again.* The fact that he used the word "we"—confirming that we had and would continue to go through my health issues as a family—meant the world to me, and helped me to face giving up my ovaries with real serenity. I scheduled a hysterectomy immediately and, *poof*, my peace of mind was fully restored.

This was a very personal decision, not made lightly, and I am not in any way saying it is the right decision for every woman. There are alternatives, as I've already indicated. These consist, primarily, of drugs that are, most often, taken after the facts of chemo, radiation, and surgery, in cases where the cancer is hormone-receptor-positive, and that in some biochemical way work to block the effects of your body's estrogen on your body. What are the drugs I'm talking about and how do they work?

- Selective estrogen receptor response modulators (SERMs). SERMs work by blocking the effects estrogen has on breast tissue. They do this by attaching to the estrogen receptors—specific protein molecules within the cell—so that estrogen itself will be unable to attach to the cell and tell it to grow. One of the most common SERMS prescribed for breast cancer treatment is Tamoxifen, and another is Fareston, though this latter is often used in cases of more advanced cancers for women who are post-menopausal.

- Estrogen receptor downregulators (ERDs). ERDs also block the effects of estrogen on the cell by attaching to the estrogen receptors, but they also both reduce the number of estrogen receptors in the cell and change the actual shape of the receptors so that estrogen can't attach to them as efficiently. ERDs are most commonly used in cases of hormone-receptor-positive breast cancer when the cancer is in an advanced stage, the patient is post-menopausal, and other hormone therapy medications, such as Tamoxifen, are no longer doing the job.

- Aromatase inhibitors. These drugs, which include brand names like Arimidex, Fermara, and Aromasin, work by stopping the production of estrogen, and are used only for post-menopausal women. This is because aromatase inhibitors don't impact the ovaries—and because the ovaries in post-menopausal women have already, naturally stopped producing estrogen and the main source of estrogen in their bodies comes from fat and the adrenal glands. These drugs stop the production of estrogen by blocking aromatase, a naturally occurring enzyme, from turning the hormone androgen into estrogen, so even less estrogen is available to trigger cancer cell growth.

● **Luteinizing hormone-releasing hormone agents (LHRHs).** LHRHs, on the other hand, do work on the ovaries—they shut them down so they produce no estrogen, and less total estrogen is then available in the body to impact the growth of cancer cells. These drugs can be used on pre-menopausal women with early-stage breast cancer because when the medicines are stopped, the ovaries begin to work again, although how long it will take for any individual woman's ovaries to recover will vary. LHRHs are given by injection, often on a monthly basis; brand names include Lupron, Trelstar, and Zoladex.

If hormone-receptor-positive cancers do not respond to the treatments listed above, there are other drugs that a doctor can recommend. Halotestin, for example, which is an anabolic steroid and helps to reduce the amount of estrogen in the body, or Magace, a form of progestin that suppresses the effect estrogen has on breast cancer cells.

What are the risks of hormonal therapies like these? Well, each of these drugs can trigger side effects—nausea, vomiting, diarrhea or constipation, hot flashes, headaches, fluid retention and swelling, bone pain and/or increased bone loss, fatigue, skin rashes, and weight gain are common ones. Even though these side effects are, at best, unpleasant, often, depending on the other methods used to treat breast cancer, these drugs make sense as part of a total cancer treatment program because of their relative toxicity, when compared with chemotherapy or radiation therapy. The real reason for concern regarding these drugs is that, while they may help to cure breast cancer and/or help to keep breast cancer from recurring, they may, themselves, trigger the development of other cancers such as ovarian or endometrial.[144] As with most methods of treating breast cancer—from chemo to radiation to surgery and now to hormonal therapy—each patient has to weigh the potential benefits against the potential detriments, balance these pros and cons with the specifics of her individual, unique manifestation of cancer, and decide for herself what treatments make sense.

For me, a hysterectomy made the most sense. And, frankly, I was grateful to have my periods go away. I had not been menopausal at the time of my diagnosis, but I had, even previ-

---

144 http://www.thelancet.com/journals/lancet/article/PIIS0140-6736(89)91141-0/abstract.

ous to that diagnosis, actually looked forward to having one less thing to fuss about every month. I suppose I consider the end of my periods to be one of the good things to have come out of my cancer experience.

Now, keeping all this in mind, the subject of hormones comes down to two dramatically opposed concepts to consider. On one hand, we know that hormones influence the growth of cancer. If your cancer is hormone positive, estrogen feeds it—and whether you are post- or pre-menopausal, your body is producing this estrogen in some quantity, somewhere—in your ovaries, adrenal gland, fat tissue. Doctors often recommend trying to 'remedy' this production by way of drugs or surgery.

On the other hand—and this really is in direct contrast to the idea of a 'remedy' for estrogen—estrogen is good for us. It helps to prevent bone loss, weight gain, and the growth of facial hair. It helps to keep our libidos in good working order. It helps us maintain a sense of balance, both mental balance—lubricating our brains to think and remember, and evening out mood swings—and physical balance. Remember that old commercial with an elderly man or woman uttering the tag line, "Help, I've fallen and I can't get up"? A lack of hormones—estrogen for her and testosterone for him—has likely played a part in their inability to stay upright. I had one patient, a twenty-five-year-old man, who was otherwise in excellent health, tell me he felt "off balance" all of the time—while playing basketball, walking to work, driving his car. The answer to his problem was just one blood test away: he had a very low testosterone level. Supplementing with testosterone-increasing supplements, because he wanted the most natural approach possible, worked well and gave him his balance—his confidence, and his life—back.

Let me mention at this juncture, however, that almost nothing gets under my skin like the general acceptance within the medical, and social, communities that, if something goes wrong in a woman's life once she hits her 40s, it "must be hormones." The cause of whatever problem she is presenting with *can* be hormones, but it is a pet peeve of mine that most doctors will not take the time to figure out what else it could be. It is just "easier" to prescribe an antidepressant for her, or recommend hormone replacement therapy (HRT)—which itself, as we all know by now, has been tied incontrovertibly to the development of cancer. To this I say, *Easier for whom?* Hormones have a big influence on our lives, but they are not omnipotent. Say a woman tells her doctor she's frequently feeling sad or angry, and she traces the emotions to dissatisfaction in her marriage. The dissatisfaction could be because her hormones are unbalanced. It could also be because her husband's a jackass and the right thing to do would be to find that out before you medicate her.

With apologies to Shakespeare: To take hormones (HRT) or to block hormones—that is the question. There is a great deal of gray area here, neither path cheerfully without hazard, so the call is a difficult one.

Personally, I will not give a moment's thought to hormone replacement in any form and, because I'm also trying to avoid estrogenic foods, I'm working on natural ways to block estrogen uptake with things like ipriflavone. But many people, depending on their own hormone receptor status, can safely try to help themselves with menopausal symptoms using alternative approaches. These alternatives can include food and herbs as well as supplements. I'm going to give you a rather comprehensive list of what is available, but I caution you that, if you have or have had hormone-receptive-positive cancer, you will want to be careful with the remedies that are pro-estrogen or pro-progesterone. Additionally, consult your doctor or pharmacist before you incorporate one of these natural remedies into your routine—natural remedies work the same way chemical ones do, by altering your body's biochemistry, and there may be interactions with medications that need to be avoided. For example, you should not take dong quai if you are on Coumadin, which is used to slow blood clotting, because dong quai can also slow blood clotting.

Herbs and Foods

- **Black Cohosh** is a phytoestrogen, or plant-based estrogen, that is useful for a range of menopausal symptoms including hot flashes, mood swings, and vaginal dryness.

- **Black current oil** is a source of gamma-linolenic acid that can influence prostaglandin synthesis, which can help soothe menopausal symptoms. This fatty acid is not something that will enhance estrogen or progesterone uptake or synthesis.

- **Dong quai,** a plant whose root is used in Chinese medicine, is not estrogenic; however, it may help support the natural balance of hormones. Note: dong quai should not be used if a woman is experiencing a heavy menstrual flow.

- **Evening primrose oil** is also a source of gamma-linolenic acid that can influence prostaglandin synthesis, which can help soothe menopausal symptoms. Another fatty acid, primrose oil is not something that will enhance estrogen or progesterone uptake or synthesis.

- **Flax seeds** are an estrogenic food. Try grinding a small handful in a coffee grinder and sprinkling them over your morning yogurt, or a salad. Never cook flax seeds as the heat destroys their nutrients.

- **Ginseng** helps to keep the vaginal walls healthy and supple, to prevent drying and tearing. It is also useful in relieving hot flashes, mood swings, and trouble sleeping. A very interesting herb, ginseng appears to be a phytoestrogen, but when carefully studied, does not appear to have estrogenic effect. That leaves us without a good answer as to whether or not we should be using it if we have an estrogen-positive cancer

- **Soy** is another phytoestrogen. Fermented soy products such as tempeh or miso paste, as a seasoning, are preferred over non-fermented. Remember to eat only organic soy products that don't contain any GMO soy.

- **Wild Yam** helps to regulate hormones, especially progesterone. It is something that would be considered a natural progesterone replacement, so if you have a progesterone-positive cancer, think carefully about the pros and cons as you make a personalized decision.

- **There are many other** estrogenic foods including olives, sunflower seeds, papaya, garlic, beets, licorice, plums, cherries, carrots, tomatoes, peas, parsley, sage, eggs, dates and apples; you may want to incorporate more of these whole foods into your diet.

Supplements

- **Melatonin** is one of my personal favorite remedies. This compound, found naturally in feverfew and St. John's wort but which can be purchased as a supplement in pill form, is a godsend in dealing with insomnia. Interestingly though, too high a dose could give you some B-grade horror-movie nightmares, so start with a low dose and work up gradually.

- **Vitamin E,** among its many other benefits, can help alleviate hot flashes.

- **Vitamin B** complex is wonderful for counterbalancing stress.

At the end of the day, the hard questions about hormones remain for all women, and they are even more complicated for cancer survivors. We answer them differently, depending on our age when we were diagnosed, if we have already had our children, and other personal priorities. For most of us, the dilemma comes down to wondering how to paint a Monet when we have no pink left on our palette. How do we make ourselves look, and feel, the same as we did before we got cancer?

The reality is that, after cancer, we are not the same people we were before we battled the disease. The crucible of cancer changes us mentally, spiritually, and physically. The challenge is to find new ways to love our lives and our new selves, and sex may be the perfect metaphor in this case. For some people—for most people—the act of making love after breast cancer is going to require a different and heightened level of trust with your partner, a different and hard-earned confidence in yourself, a willingness to think creatively, differently, and break old habits in order to find new ways to express your passion. If you have no yellow on your palette, it doesn't mean you can't paint a beautiful painting, but it will be a different painting than the one you would have painted with that color available to you.

Different, but no less a masterpiece.

12

Ahhhhh! Massage, Meditation, and a Little Math

Getting a massage is not a passive experience.

Julie

Like all good authors, Ankit and I
have saved the best revelation for last: you, as a breast cancer
patient and, ultimately, as a breast cancer survivor, get a lifetime pass to have as many massages as you like. For most of
us—me included—massage has been a wonderful treat, a
reward when we have worked out every day for a month or a
special indulgence when we're on vacation. During and after
breast cancer, however, massage becomes an essential part of
your recovery, as well as the maintenance, of your health. Why?
Let's start with a few of the reasons we've already touched on
and cover them in a bit more detail.

Lymphatic Drainage

Your lymphatic system is, to boil it down to a concept we can
easily visualize, a series of ducts and drains that function as a
sort of human septic system. This is the system that drains tox-

ins and waste products from your body, and the benefits of getting the lymph fluid flowing and moving through and out of the body more quickly and efficiently are myriad. Some people are interested in the technique simply as a beauty treatment—it can help to reduce the appearance of cellulite, and reduce the skin inflammation we commonly call acne. For breast cancer patients and survivors, the stakes become higher.

- **Lymphatic drainage massage** can reduce the swelling and discomfort of lymphedema, and even prevent it altogether—an exquisite reason for mastectomy patients, especially those who have also had lymph nodes surgically removed, to avail themselves of the treatment.

- **Lymphatic drainage can** also help mastectomy patients in that, by draining fluid from the site of wounds on the breast tissue, where scars are typically formed, it enhances the ability of the tissue to reconstruct itself and thereby help the wound to heal with less scarring.

- **Lymphatic drainage helps** to push the toxic chemicals or free radicals that come with chemotherapy and/or radiation treatments through the system and so cleanse the body.

During the time immediately before and after my surgery, I was absolutely religious about my massage schedule, though having massages as often as I liked to have them, and as was warranted by both my chemo and my surgery, was a strain on the family budget. So I'll let you in on a little secret: you can do lymphatic massage on yourself. I often did this in between my sessions with my massage therapist.

Lymphatic drainage massage is a very slow and gentle massage technique. Start by reaching up to your neck and placing the four fingers of each hand on the soft tissue just above your collarbone. Place the little finger of your left hand in the hollow just to the left of your throat and line the other fingers up beside it, just above the collarbone; do the same on your right side with your right hand. Very slowly and gently, begin to "pump" in a small downward motion. Do this about twenty times. This activates the lymph fluid so it begins to move. You might actually feel the fluid start to move, in most cases in your throat or in the pressure inside your ear.

The fluid in the breasts—the fluid we want to drain—moves in a circular pattern around the nipple area and upward into your armpit. Place your fingers flat at the top of your breast and move your hand around your breast—again, slowly and gently—going from the top, to the inside, then the underside of your breast, drawing your hand up toward your armpit. The motion you'll want to make runs clockwise on your right breast, and counterclockwise for your left. Do this to one breast about twenty times.

When you have completed those twenty strokes for one breast, take your opposite hand and use your middle finger to find the deepest part of your armpit. Press this place with steady, gentle pressure for about twenty seconds; then repeat the process for your other breast. Repeat the exercise two or three times a day.

Range of Motion

As I've already said, working on maintaining, and even improving your range of motion—how far above your head or behind your body you can reach with your arm—is important to do *before and after* you have your surgery. This is because scar tissue wants to contract as it heals, and it actually never wants to stop contracting. But our bodies are designed to expand! Stop and take a deep breath right now. Feel how your chest, your back, and even your arm muscles if you are breathing deeply enough, will expand to accommodate the breath. Stretching your chest and arm muscles through yoga or other exercise is critical to maintaining comfort after your surgery, including comfort in the simple act of breathing.

For me, being able to fill my chest without restriction has allowed me to continue, post-surgery, to take part in one of the most fulfilling and relaxing "extracurricular" activities on my schedule: singing in my church choir. I'm able to take in enough air to hold a note as long as I could before my surgery—before all this new scar tissue was a part of my chest area. Not a big deal for those of you who don't sing? Keeping your chest muscles stretched and supple allows your lungs, and your heart, the room they need to expand, so your capacity to perform nearly every activity of life is enhanced—to make it around the mall on a shopping trip without having to sit to catch your breath, to play a game of pick-up basketball with your son without gasping, to enjoy lovingly prolonged love making.

I also believe—and this is an intuitive understanding, not something your every-day surgeon is going to tell you before he operates on you—that by stretching my muscles prior to surgery, and providing Ankit the nimble muscles and expanded surface to operate on, I increased my opportunity for a good outcome. He wasn't starting out with a small, contracted foundation but, because I had steadily stretched and soothed my chest and arm area into the best shape they'd been in since my twenties, he had more surface area to work on as he transplanted my stomach fat to my breast area.

Reflexology

Reflexology, like another treatment I have mentioned in this book, acupuncture, is a bodywork technique that often gets short shift (and sometimes laughs) when you mention it as a true healing therapy. There aren't a lot of scientific studies to explain if it works, or how, so it isn't possible to recommend from a scientific, or medical standpoint. However, my opinion about it is that it will never hurt you, and it definitely feels good, so why take a pass on it? I mentioned in the Introduction that accidentally massaging my own foot in a hot bath, hitting the pressure point that reflexologists associate with breast health, made me feel good—and, indeed, inspired this book. The technique dates from the Egyptian dynastic period, so it has been around for a good long time; even if its only benefit has been to make millions of people *feel* better over thousands of years, I'm all for it.

Meditation and Creative Visualization

Massage is a great way to relax, as most of us can attest—and relaxing as deeply and intently as we do when we get a massage is a beautiful way to banish unhealthy stress from our lives, at least temporarily. For cancer patients, and for survivors, I think it is important to take that natural ease we feel on a massage table to its next highest level. As I said in the quotation that opens this chapter, massage is not a passive experience. Or, in any case, it doesn't have to be one. It can be so much more if it is an event in which we are fully engaged. How?

Well, first of all, it is an opportunity to practice that *I-come-first* way of thinking. This will be especially important after your cancer treatments are over and everyone around you can see that you are healing and getting back to normal—when concern about your health is no longer their first concern, and no longer the center of your universe, either. Scheduling a regular massage means you are scheduling regular time to priori-tize your health and well being.

Your massage time is also one of the best times for you to practice creative visualization or guided imagery—the practice of positive thinking, of creating a positive outcome in your mind so that you can work toward manifesting that outcome in the real world. Personally, I don't like to talk, or for my ther-apist to do a lot of talking, while I am in the process of massage. For me, during my cancer treatment, this time was sixty or ninety minutes of holding the images of cancer cells shrivel-ing and dying off, of my scar tissue expanding with healthy, pink flexibility. It was the time when I pictured myself whole again and heading off to Greece with my children for a friend's wedding—a trip we actually got to take when I was recovered.

The healing capacity of the human body, if we give it the right tools and circumstances to do so, is astonishing. When we engage our minds in the healing, direct with intent our positive thought-energy to this goal, the capacity just might well be almost limitless.

Heart Math

When I first heard about HeartMath I thought it was the cool-est thing ever—intuitively, I understood what Doc Childre, the founder of the Institute of HeartMath, was talking about, and

I knew that the tools he was providing to help people tune into the *intelligence of the heart* were some of the most elementally important ones our modern civilization could ever discover. It is bragging a little to say it, but I was excited about Heart-Math before Fortune 500 companies like Hewlett-Packard and Motorola and all four branches of the US military decided to use HeartMath to teach their employees about emotional intelligence, mental balance, and help them to create positive transformation for themselves as individuals as well as for their companies, within the workplace.

The premise of HeartMath is to potentiate the heart's innate capacity to be the body's and the mind's conductor. How can the heart—basically a big, powerful muscle—lead over our physical bodies or our willful brains? The four basic pieces of science to understanding HeartMath are:

- **The heart sends** information neurologically to the body and the brain.

- **The heart sends** energy through the pulse, or a *blood pressure wave*. Research has demonstrated that the electrical activity of our brain changes in relation to the activity of the blood pressure wave.

- **The heart releases** a hormone called atrial peptide. This hormone inhibits the release of stress hormones. This is the heart's way of communicating, biochemically, with the rest of the body.

● **The heart also communicates** electromagnetically. When your doctor tests your heart rhythms by measuring them with an EKG, she is actually measuring the signals your heart is sending—signals that are picked up elsewhere and anywhere in the body, and that permeate the space around us so they impact us internally as well as being perceived by those who are in our space.

What does this mean in practical terms? The heart is an electrical organ, and it is wired to send *out* its electrical pulses. Moreover, its pulses vary. That is, the heart is not a metronome; it beats faster or slower, depending on the state of mind of its owner. When its owner is, for example, angry or stressed, the heartbeat is fast, and the pulse is flat. When we are angry or stressed, we are tapping into our body's *sympathetic nervous system*, the system that triggers our fight-or-flight response. On the other hand, when we are at rest, tapped into the body's *parasympathetic nervous system*, for example after eating and while digesting, the pulse is rhythmic, and the pattern of the pulses, when mapped by scientists, make beautiful patterns. HeartMath teaches us how to locate that place of rest and peace, and *live* there.

And not only that—not only can we train ourselves to generate these beautiful pulses of energy, but we can train others to do so, too. Have you ever seen the joyous photographs of John Unger and his dog Shoep?[145] These two clearly shared

---

145 http://www.huffingtonpost.com/2013/08/03/schoep-tribute_n_3697248.html.

parasympathetic heart rhythms. Are you overwhelmed with a sense of ease when you and your spouse hold hands or kiss? This is because your heart rhythms have synchronized. Have you ever been in a group, in church at prayer or in a concert arena listening to a favorite musician, and you felt an unexplainable vibration of elation? This is due to the shared pulsing of your hearts. Have you ever been introduced to a total stranger and felt yourself instantly attracted to him or to her? This is likely because the electrical pulses emanating from her heart are coming from a place of peace, and you instinctively know that this person is in a place that is good. That being in this person's presence is going to be good for you.

The exercises in the HeartMath system can help you be that person who is good to be around—good for yourself as well as good for others.

13

Cancer Treatment: The Next Generation

In the 1950s, the recommended treatment for breast cancer was radical mastectomy, as well as removal of the ovaries and adrenal glands, both of which produce estrogen. In the mid-1980s, the first papers were published that noted reconstruction surgery didn't seem to interfere with recovery. By the mid-1990s, advances in both treatment protocols and diagnostic methods had changed the way we think about breast cancer, and deal with it. The advances we're making now, in 2013? If you look at where we started, what we're able to do now takes your breath away.

Ankit

If what we're able to do for breast
cancer patients now, that we weren't able to do even a few years ago, takes your breath away, where we're going is science fantasy morphed into science fact. Less than forty years ago, doctors were debating whether or not reconstruction surgery interfered with being able to beat cancer; today, two or three days every week, I perform microsurgeries to restore the look and feel of a natural breast. This may seem like a broad generalization, but it's my guess that this is the part of their jobs most doctors like the best: the constant challenge to learn new treatments and techniques to improve what we can do for our patients. In my consultation room, where I ordinarily first meet a new patient, there are several boxes of tissues in convenient locations. My patients, and often their partners and other family members, need the tissues on their first visit because there can be tears—of fear, and of anger. The leap that happens at the other end of surgery, when a patient sees her new breast or breasts for the first time—the leap of confidence, happiness, energy—that is something that is, plainly, electric.

I don't mean to suggest that breast cancer isn't a complex disease, or that its ultimate cure isn't elusive. The sense of optimism and excitement created by the on-going research and scientific breakthroughs, however, is not to be underrated.

So, what are some of the advances that have made us so enthusiastic? They currently revolve around four main areas: radiation, immunology, chemotherapy, and the study of mitochondria.

Radiation

The next generation of radiation treatment may be something called INTRABEAM® Intraoperative Radiotherapy (IORT). Currently in clinical trials, IORT may offer breast cancer patients meeting specific conditions a brand new treatment option. Traditional radiation is administered externally, and almost always following surgery. IORT differs radically from this approach: it is delivered internally, *during* surgery. That is, the surgeon performs, for example, a lumpectomy; after the surgeon has removed the tumor, the radiation oncologist immediately steps in to postion the IORT applicator in the area of the breast where the tumor had been. A single dose of radiation therapy, lasting anywhere from thirty to forty minutes, is applied; then the applicator is withdrawn and the surgeon closes the incision. This is in contrast to traditional, external-beam radiation in which once-daily radiation sessions are employed for six weeks. IORT, as I said, is still in clinical trials, and it is not, so far, suggested that it is a replacement for traditional radiation, but rather a method of administering a direct and concentrated dose of radiation to the immediately affected tissues, with less potential for radiation damage to surrounding healthy tissue.

Immunology

Immunology is the branch of biomedical science that focuses on the body's immune system. So, what is the immune system? Think of it as the body's alarm system. As the name suggests, it isn't just one part of the body, in just one place, though 70 to 80% of it is located in the gut area; it is a network of cells, tissues, and organs throughout the body that work together to defend against dangerous intruders. These intruders can be harmful bacteria, fungi, parasites, or other microscopic organisms. It is the immune system's job to keep them out or, should the invaders breech the system, to then kill them.

When the immune system detects an invading microorganism, it mobilizes an elegantly complex and elaborate communications system throughout the body to alert millions and millions of different sorts of cells to begin to produce powerful biochemicals that regulate the behavior and growth of the invaders in order to destroy them. If you looked at the body's counterattack under a microscope, you might think it resembled an NFL defensive line play—only multiplied by several hundred thousand times the players.

When the immune system's defensive line fails to block the opposing advance, however, a wide range of disorders and diseases, from allergic reactions to diabetes, to autoimmune disease and cancer—are the result.

Given the importance of a healthy immune system to our on-going health, science still knows relatively little about it. What we are learning is that suppressing the system in order to fight disease is the wrong course. Rather, we need to regulate and rebalance this system, keep it in good working order, to *prevent* as well as to defeat disease. When it comes specifically to cancer, however, things are a little more—what else is new—complicated. In this case, not only does the immune system need to be in good balance and ready to defend the body, the immune system has to be educated about how to find the invaders it must defend against. The problem, you see, is that cancer cells aren't *outside* invaders, they are our body's own cells—mutated and malignant, but nevertheless our own. Because they are our own cells, they are often not different enough from the typical invader cell for the immune system to react to them and attack. Researchers are currently developing clinical trials to study new immune-based therapies—including therapeutic vaccinations for various cancers, such as breast cancer. Unlike typical vaccines, which are given to supposedly *prevent* disease, cancer vaccines boost the body's immune system so it has a greater capacity to go on attack against formerly hard-to-discern cancer cells.

Another exciting advancement being made in the field of immunology concerns identifying tumor targets, known as *antigens*, and aiming antibodies at them. That is, scientists are finding ways to use chemicals to target not the whole cancer cell, but specific biochemicals—specifically DNA biochemicals—that are produced only within the cancer cell. Again, let's use a football analogy: this method of treatment is like running a play in which no other member of the lineup is touched, but the quarterback is sacked, and sacked good. In the late 1990s, the first of these therapeutic antibodies was approved to treat breast cancer—Herceptin. Herceptin works by attaching itself to the HER2 receptors on the cancer cell and, so, blocks it from receiving growth signals.

Other biologic therapies available for women who have advanced, or metastasized HER2-positive breast cancer, include a drug called Tykerb, which works by interfering with certain specific proteins in the cancer cells that cause it to divide and grow in a rapid, abnormal way, and a drug called Femara, which works by inhibiting the enzyme that releases estrogen from fat.

The scientific community is not only developing new and more targeted drugs, however; it is also working on an exciting new way to deliver the drugs: *nanoparticles*. Nanoparticles are currently an area of intense scientific interest. A nanoparticle, which can be in a powder, a cluster, or a crystal form, is, by definition, a microscopic particle that has a dimension of less than 100 nanometers[146] on at least one of its sides. What excites scientists about this tremendously small discovery is that nanoparticles could be the bridge between bulk material and atomic structures. That is, because of the size and other characteristics of the nanoparticle, it can overcome a great many of the limitations of the current ways in which we deliver drugs. For example, because of these characteristics, a nanoparticle has increased circulation in the bloodstream. Nanoparticles also have the ability to be accumulated within a cell without triggering drug resistance. Using nanoparticles, then, to deliver chemo drugs can result in the better targeting of *just* cancer cells.

Chemotherapy

For a long time, there have been influential people in the oncology community who have been telling patients not to use antioxidants when they are undergoing chemotherapy. Intuitively, Julie told me, she thought this was incorrect—if free radicals help to *cause* cancer, wouldn't reducing the free radicals in our systems help to cure cancer? So, when she was diagnosed with breast cancer and decided that chemo would need to be part of her treatment, she was very motivated to

---

146 How big is a nanometer? A meter is 39 inches long—and a nanometer is *one-billionth* of a meter.

look into this subject. She understood that some of her chemo agents specifically required oxidative stress to be present for the few short hours it was actively killing cancer cells, but what she found on a broader level was that the National Institutes of Health itself disagreed with the naysayers. Quite the contrary, what the NIH had to say was that not only did antioxidants generally *not* interfere with the efficacy of chemotherapy drugs, antioxidants actually *decreased* the side effects of chemo drugs by protecting healthy tissue in the body from their effects, and they *enhanced* the killing capacity of the drugs on cancer cells, and patients who took antioxidants during chemo actually had increased survival rates.[147] Indeed, the next generation of chemotherapy drugs may *be* antioxidants.

Mitochondria

Another area of interest in the on-going quest to understand and defeat cancer is the *mitochondria*. The mitochondria are structures within our cells that act as power plants because they generate *adenosine triphosphate*, or ATP, which is the source of a cell's chemical energy. A more apt analogy than "power plants" might be "oil refineries"—that is, as a car uses gasoline created from various forms of crude oil, the mitochondria

---

147 http://www.ncbi.nlm.nih.gov/pubmed/17283738.

manufacture ATP from the sources of nutrition—carbs, proteins and fats—that we provide them.

So what do the mitochondria have to do with cancer? Well, that's what researchers are trying to figure out. It is easy, however, to understand *why* they're interested in this particular atomic structure: low muscle tone and fatigue are part of many diseases; dysfunctional mitochondria result in low muscle tone and fatigue; mitochondrial dysfunction is the result of oxidative stress which is, itself, as we now know, a part of many diseases. It's not hard to follow the bouncing ball on this problem.

What is fascinating is that we are learning to optimize mitochondrial function with very special attention to diet, by implementing a *ketogenic* diet. The ketogenic diet—high in fats, adequate in protein, and low in carbs—probably benefits us in several ways. It imitates starvation by providing very little carbohydrate—and calorie reduction helps with weight loss overall, something most of us need. The other thing that occurs with carbohydrate, and by extension, sugar reduction, that is a specific benefit for cancer patients, is that cancer cells that love to feed on glucose are deprived of their preferred fuel source, and they are more likely to die. In addition to significantly reducing carbohydrate and sugar, a ketogenic diet provides just the right amount of protein, limiting our overconsumption of animal proteins, another thing that is likely to be an anticancer approach. The balance of the ketogenic diet, with its limited carbs and protein, is consumed as fat, with a focus on healthy fats, such as those from nuts and seeds. When our mitochondria are provided with healthy fat, they are able to work far more optimally to produce ATP, our cells' gasoline, than they do with any other fuel source. While achieving ketosis is a tremendous challenge for the patient following a ketogenic diet, metabolic ketosis is showing great potential as another tool to add to our cancer treatment toolbox.

One of the things that should be obvious as you've read through this breakthrough and "what's on the horizon" chapter is that some of the focus of treatment is making radical shifts. Rather than looking for a slightly new version of an old technique or an already existing class of chemotherapy, we're looking at cancer with fresh eyes, focusing on antioxidants, helping the immune system to help itself, and paying much more attention to food—which may well be our most important medicine.

We may be coming to a point in health care where we no longer view a diagnosis of cancer as a battle not to die, but as an opportunity to improve our health. And we really do know how to do it, too: eating good, whole foods that are rich in antioxidants, taking appropriate dietary supplements, being regularly physically active, and reducing our daily stress load.

Conclusion

Our Exceptional Sorority

It is harder to be a cancer survivor
than it is to be a cancer patient.

Julie

Let me say that again: It is harder to

be a cancer survivor than it is to be a cancer patient.

It just is, and I will tell you why: in the absence of recurrent treatments, fresh scars, and generally feeling like crap pretty much twenty-four hours a day, it is all too easy to forget how rigorous you need to be to maintain the health you got back.

Taking an integrative, functional approach to health isn't easy—especially not in a world that doesn't embrace it. We live in a culture where we can be watching TV and an advertisement for McDonald's French fries (a food-like product that clogs our arteries, plays havoc with our cholesterol, and causes us to be fat) is followed by an advertisement for a drug that helps keep our arteries clear, lowers our cholesterol, or helps us lose weight. If there is a pill to cure it, why worry about giving ourselves the disease? We can just get the doc to write a prescription after we're diagnosed!

It is far too easy to lose the discipline we impose on ourselves during our treatment when, once again, we are feeling fine. We have to find ways to continue to remind ourselves of the lessons cancer has taught us.

For me this has meant coming to grips with the fact that my passion for doing as much as I can, for packing every minute of the day with an activity, has not diminished. I like chasing life as if I'm wearing a pair of roller blades and my hair is on fire—this is who I am; I am still at my most joy-filled when I am rolling at this speed.

The difference is that, these days, when the activity or the speed of it doesn't feel right—when it is causing me stress rather than joy—I fix it. Immediately. My response to stress these days is not to grit my teeth and power through it, but to drop back into a position of self-care. I don't direct all of my energy out into the world anymore; these days, I save some of it for me. I take walks on the beach with my kids and the dog. I make time to walk, and to take regular yoga classes. I get a massage at least every other week. I sit down to dinner with my family. I go to my favorite shop after work and buy myself a pretty new blouse to wear at that weekend's speaking engagement, or I go to the mall to purchase the new curtains I want for the family room.

How do I manage to do these things—and not feel guilty? What are some of the coping tools I use to redirect the energy?

Foremost is, simply, to think about my family. My husband and my two children are my highest priority—and I remind myself that by taking care of me, I am taking care of them. By maintaining my health and my happiness, I am creating the healthy, happy wife and mother they deserve.

Having cancer is similar to having autism, which was my first specialty. This idea might feel like a stretch, so hear me out. Prior to my daughter's autism diagnosis, my pediatric practice was a fairly typical, American one, featuring annual well-child check-ups. When Dani was diagnosed, however, I immediately started walking a different path—learning about autism and how to help Dani heal her body, including her brain, so she could have the happiest and most productive life possible. This is all any parent can ask for any child, but when autism is in the picture, you have to find a different way to happiness, and you have to find it quickly.

Moreover, you will find very few people whose lives don't include autism, who will have any clue what the scenery along that path looks like. This is one of the reasons you will find that, among the parents of autistic children, the bond is tight. We know what each other have been going through, and will be going through. We can share war stories, treatment successes, and pain—and we can laugh together at things that might make folks without autism in the family squeamish.

The same is true of having breast cancer. When it becomes part of our lives, we are immediately shaken off that path we have been on and we have to find a new way to travel. The good news is that we immediately become part of an exclusive sorority—other women who have or have had breast cancer, too. I like to think of us as steel magnolias, we women who have walked this hard breast cancer path together.

This does not mean that each of us has chosen the same treatment or the same reconstruction option. Far from it. We are all different women—our ages are different, our life circumstances are different, our cancers are different.

What we have in common is that we have all been called on to summon the physical, mental, emotional, and spiritual fortitude it takes to face, and beat, breast cancer. Our physical, mental, emotional, and spiritual shapes have been forever altered by our encounter with this disease. We can share war stories, treatment successes, and pain—and we can laugh together at things that might make folks without breast cancer in the family squeamish, and do it with a sense of humor that has been tempered in the crucible.

Being a cancer survivor is harder than being a cancer patient because we have learned that we can never again take our health for granted. I have often said that cancer is the best thing that ever happened to me. It has allowed me to focus on things that bring me joy, that nourish and sustain me. These are lessons we all encourage each other to learn, but finding myself on the doorstep of the school called cancer made it a lot easier to go to class and take those lessons to heart. The trick is in remembering those lessons every day, no matter how far down the road of health and survivorship I may journey. My prayer is that the same will be true for each of you who read this book. In starting here, may you be well on the way to health and healing!

Resources

Cookbooks

Food is our most important medicine. Our diet is the first line of defense when it comes to our health. The nutrients in apples and spinach, eggs and chicken, rice and quinoa empower our bodies to function efficiently on a cellular level—when our cells are healthy, our whole bodies are healthy; when our cells, or components of our cells, are not healthy, we are sick, *but we can help to restore glowing good health by giving our cells the nutrients they need to heal.* So. When I was diagnosed with cancer, I knew food was going to be a big part of my recovery. But I was not interested in using food to survive. I was interested in using food as another tool to beat my cancer. As I looked at the plethora of cookbooks that are out there, I was struck by the fact that their titles seem to speak volumes—and that helped to guide me toward the books I needed.

The Cancer Fighting Kitchen[1] by Rebecca Katz and Mat Edelson (Ten Speed Press, 2010) became my favorite title. It is more than a simple cookbook. It contains information on the healing qualities of different foods and herbs, and the authors discuss the importance of eating organic in a way

---

1 http://www.amazon.com/The-Cancer-Fighting-Kitchen-Nourishing-Big-Flavor-ebook/dp/B004477UG2/ref=tmm_kin_title_popover?ie=UTF8&qid=1381 871169&sr=8-1

that is understandable and provokes action. They also talk about seasoning food to make meals that are not just palatable but delicious for people who are going through chemo and/or radiation, when things don't taste normal. The authors' approach is to focus on nourishing the reader, not just feeding us—and on giving us the know-how to nurture ourselves. They teach the FASS technique—that is *F*at (as olive oil), *A*cid (as lemon juice), Salt (as sea salt), and *S*weet (as organic maple syrup), or the four components of foods that contribute to both their taste and their mouth-feel and are necessary to creating meals that satisfy. Recipes are grouped by dish type rather than by what symptom they might relieve and are not restricted to a single diet. What I mean by that is, although most of the recipes are gluten free, and dairy is relatively limited as well, the authors aren't advocating for the GFCF lifestyle or the Paleo Diet or eating by blood type. Ms. Katz is a chef at a high-end restaurant, so be forewarned that a recipe might have many ingredients, but the cooking instructions are thorough, and each recipe is accompanied by enticing, beautiful photographs so you know what the end-result is supposed to look like. Even post-cancer, I still use this book regularly, especially when entertaining guests!

One Bite At A Time (Celestial Arts, 2011) is the second cookbook by Rebecca Katz and Mat Edelson, and it's filled with even more scrumptious recipes geared toward survivorship.

The Cancer Survival Cookbook: 200 Quick and Easy Recipes with Helpful Eating Hints[1] by Christina Marino and Donna L. Weihofen (Wiley, 2nd edition, 2004) is less about an approach to nutrition and nourishing yourself and more about reacting to the consequences of treatment. The language is quite conservative and the authors are not well informed about herbal approaches to nutrition or how to use supplements as part of an overall diet strategy. There are also, alas, no photographs of the prepared recipes. These things being said, this book may be valuable to people for whom using food as medicine is a new or difficult concept. The part about this book I like the most is that it breaks down the symptoms of cancer treatment and gives advice about which foods might best alleviate those symptoms including, importantly, weight loss, with helpful hints about how to incorporate more calories in recipes.

The *Betty Crocker Living with Cancer Cookbook* (Betty Crocker, 2001) features traditional, easy-to-make recipes that are not necessarily focused on nourishing the patient as much as getting calories into her. The latest edition (2011[2]) includes personal stories, nutrition tips, and quotes from breast cancer survivors, which can be inspirational to those of us in the process of recovery, and recipes that address particular symptoms are flagged.

---

1 http://www.amazon.com/The-Cancer-Survival-Cookbook-Recipes/dp/0471346683

2 http://www.amazon.com/Crocker-Living-Cancer-Cookbook-ebook/dp/B00BS03S6Y/ref=sr_1_1?ie=UTF8&qid=1383609673&sr=8-1&keywords=the+betty+crocker+living+with+cancer+cookbook

Glutathione

Glutathione is the body's own super, master, Jedi Knight anti-oxidant; supplementing the body's natural supply of it can elementally enhance recovery. Glutathione can be delivered in several ways but, whatever your method of delivery, it's critical to ensure that your supply of it has not been exposed to light or air as these have the potential to diminish glutathione's ability to reduce oxidative stress. Glutathoine can be taken:

● Intravenously

This method has to be done under the supervision of a physician, and offices that do these sorts of infusions will be largely those practicing functional or integrative medicine. See "Doctors" in this resource section for help in locating a functional medicine specialist near you.

● Transdermally

Glutathione is not easily absorbed through the skin, and the cream or lotion really has to be prepared by a good compounding pharmacy in order for this delivery method to work. Just mixing the glutathione in oil is not sufficient. One compounder that seems to have worked on transdermal meds with a good degree of success is Lee Silsby in Cleveland, Ohio. The supplement in this form, like that used in an intravenous delivery system, requires a prescription from a physician.

● Orally

There are several preparations that are precursors or combinations of antioxidants that a patient can take by mouth. I have used them in my practice. Two of my favorites are EnduraCell and Recancostat. EnduraCell is made from broccoli sprouts and not only helps the body to make glutathione, it helps the immune system to balance and function more appropriately. Recancostat is combined with several herbs that optimize glutathione synthesis.

● Inhalation via Nebulizer

With this method, the glutathione is delivered by way of the patient inhaling, and uses the IV form of the supplement delivered via a nebulizer. This method is wonderfully helpful to some people with chronic sinuses, allergies, and asthma. It does require a prescription, and be sure, once you have opened the glutathione packet, to use it immediately so it doesn't oxidize and lose its potential as an antioxidant.

Hyperbaric Chambers

There are several ways to access a hyperbaric chamber to use during your recovery. As you begin your search for a facility near you, know that hyperbaric chambers are medical equipment and, in commercial, clinical settings, must be prescribed for your use. It is exceedingly rare to find multi-place hospital-based hyperbaric chambers to use for "off-label" purposes, and they are usually very expensive. There are, however, in cities all around the country, private centers or physicians' offices with the smaller, portable, lower-pressure chambers and they often offer packages for multiple sessions or "dives". Their use is never covered by insurance except for highly specific diagnoses, none of which include cancer or the side effects of treatment, except for bone loss of the jaw associated with radiation.

Some patients may want to rent a chamber for the duration of cancer treatment. Having a chamber in your own home allows convenient, unlimited use of the chamber for a set fee over a set period of time. Often a lease can be arranged on a month-by-month basis. Other patients will want to purchase a chamber; this can be costly, but if it is within your options, a hyperbaric chamber—well cared-for—can be an important factor in maintaining the health of the person for whom the chamber was prescribed for a long time.

In all of these cases, you may find yourself on the Internet, searching to make arrangements for hyperbaric therapy. I have found, over the years, that if I'm looking for a center or a chamber just about anywhere in the country, I can call Bill Schindler in Atlanta at Hyperbaric People Helping People.[1] He has been working in the field for years and knows where most chambers are located around the country. Bill can help

---

[1] www.hyperbaricphp.com

with all things hyperbaric, or help you find someone who can if he can't.

Products

To cure cancer, and to help *prevent* cancer or the recurrence of cancer, you need to reduce your body's chemical exposure. A wonderful (if also horrifying) resource to help do this is the Environmental Working Group web site.[2] This organization rates the ingredients in many commonly available products in terms of their potential toxicities. The lower the score, the better. Some specific products I highly recommend are listed below.

Personal Products

- **Eye Drops.** Similasan Original Swiss Formula Homeopathic Dry Eye Relief has been a godsend to many women during radiation therapy. Don't let the word 'homeopathic' in the name make you think this product is hard to come by—Walmart carries it.

- **Sunscreen.** Sunscreen is important for so many reasons—from preventing the development of skin cancers to preventing premature aging from sun damage; for

---

2 www.ewg.org

women undergoing radiation therapy, or who have lost their hair during chemo, sunscreen is no longer in anyway an optional cosmetic. That being said, there is a real balancing act between getting enough Vitamin D3 through sunshine kissing your skin, and making sure not to get burned. I like MDSolarSciences Mineral Crème Broad Spectrum Sunscreen, SPF 50. It has received a '1' from the Environmental Working Group (EWG).

● **Insect repellant.** Choices are not clear in this category, and you will want to visit EWG for more options. The repellent I swear by is Ambermin; it is not listed by EWG. It is purely botanical, and I have found it to be effective in Northeast Florida where I live. As far as I know, it's available only through the Hopewell Pharmacy and Compounding Center[1] located in New Jersey.

● **Makeup.** I went looking for organic makeup right after I was diagnosed and was appalled to find what kinds of things were in most makeup products. Not every product out there has been tested by EWG, but many have, and I found Coastal Classic Creations.[2] The folks there were extremely helpful. A service representative called me back promptly after I left a message. I already felt lousy from chemo when we talked, but I described my complexion,

---

1 http://www.hopewellrx.com/category/Main-Shop-1

2 https://www.coastalclassiccreations.com

and the colors I usually wore, and the representative sent me several small trial sizes so I could make an unpressured decision. I remain a loyal customer four years later.

Appliances

Juicer. Those of us who juice can spend a lot of energy hotly debating our favored appliance. There are juicers that cut, juicers that crush, and high-speed blenders that leave all of the fiber in the drink making it less like juice and more like a smoothie. Each has its merits. A few years before I was diagnosed, I'd done research with a friend when he developed cancer and we ultimately chose a Green Star Twin Gear Juicer. For each of us, our juicer became a primary cancer fighting tool. I love the efficiency of the Green Star model I chose, and the fact that no food is wasted at all—but, let me confess, it is a pain to clean. After my first use of it—after I tasted the delicious juice it made, and knowing how nutritious this delicious drink was for my sick body—I made a commitment to clean the machine the instant I finished using it. Every single time I used it. I've developed the habit of practicing gratitude-based thinking as I clean it and using the time in this way really does make it less of a pain.

Household Products

From no Volatile Organic Compound (VOC) paint to organic cleaning products to enviro-friendly building materials, entire books can and have been written on what to look for when building, remodeling or just living in your home. It's important to understand that a *green* home isn't necessarily a healthy home. Similarly, a *sustainable* home or a *natural* home isn't necessarily a healthy home. Why? Well, if you buy a product that brags about its all-natural ingredients, you would do well to remember that arsenic is natural and you don't want arsenic in your shampoo or dishwashing liquid any more than you want arsenic in your paint or arsenic residue in the fabric in which your sofa is upholstered.

The idea of healthy living includes using cleaning and building products that will actually promote health. This is a cornerstone of the HealthyUNow Foundation's approach. The Foundation's web site,[1] is still under construction as I write this in October of 2013, but it will eventually be a resource that will help people to make healthier choices as they build, remodel, or redecorate—or simply keep clean—their home. There are, increasingly, numbers of healthy building and healthy living consultants who can help with construction projects, choosing the least problematic materials for your remodel or build—people like Anthony Brenner, who is a part of our Bird's Nest project at the HealthyUNow Foundation; access Anthony through the HealthyUNow Foundation site. In the meantime,

---

1 www.healthyunow.org

there are other resources to help you sort through what you might want to change to make your home healthier.[2]

As trees are the 'lungs' of the earth, so plants can be the 'lungs' of a home. Keep in mind that plants are an excellent way to help detoxify your home as well.[3]

Exercise

As I hope we made clear in this book, exercise is something you simply cannot do without if you hope to remain healthy—strong, flexible, and vibrant. A good program includes a variety of exercises that focus on three different, foundational aspects of physical health: cardio, strength training, and stretching.

The National Institute of Health, through the National Institute on Aging, has an excellent online guide to exercise.[4] While this program is geared for seniors, it also, in my opinion, offers very fine guidelines for every age, and it is an excellent place to start for those who might have led a lifestyle that was fairly sedentary and are just beginning to get back into a regular exercise routine.

---

2   http://www.ewg.org/guides/cleaners and http://www.ewg.org/research/healthy-home-tips/tip-14-your-healthy-home-checklist

3   http://www.greenyour.com/home/lawn-garden/houseplant/tips/choose-plants-that-purify-the-indoor-air

4   http://www.nia.nih.gov/health/publication/exercise-physical-activity/introduction

Cancer Fitness: Exercise Programs for Patients and Survivors[1] by Anna Schwartz (Touchstone, 2004) is an excellent resource for developing your own cancer, and post-cancer, workout. I like the author's point that often cancer patients believe that rest is going to help them most of all toward their goal of wellness. While the appropriate amount and quality of sleep is critical to recovery, it is not *all* we cancer patients and survivors need: without the appropriate amount and quality of physical activity, we grow even more weak and fatigued—too weak and fatigued to give cancer our best fight.

Mark Huston, MD, wrote a book called *What Your Doctor May Not Tell You About Heart Disease* (Grand Central, 2012).[2] This book has a fabulous chapter on exercise—vigorous, rigorous exercise—and it is very detailed in how to go about it. Huston's program may be too much for most of us while we are in the thick of cancer treatment, but it is a goal to reach for!

Other Books

As I was combing through the many books I have read or need to read at my bedside table, it occurred to me that there are other books out there that offer some detailed information that

---

[1] http://www.amazon.com/Cancer-Fitness-Exercise-Survivors-ebook/dp/B0036QVOH8/ref=tmm_kin_swatch_0?_encoding=UTF8&sr=&qid=

[2] http://www.amazon.com/Doctor-about-Heart-Disease-ebook/dp/B004QZ-9PMY/ref=sr_1_2_title_0_main?s=books&ie=UTF8&qid=1382207090&sr=1-2&keywords=mark+huston+what+your+doctor+heart+disease

exceeds the scope of what we set out to do as we wrote this book.

David Servan-Schreiber, MD, PhD was a brain cancer survivor. The first time he survived, he pursued the traditional approach only. The second time he survived, he added a functional/integrative medicine approach, with a much healthier and longer lasting remission. He ultimately lost his battle with brain cancer in 2011, and the last work he focused on was the way cell phones and EMF (Electric and Magnetic Fields) were contributing to causing cancer. He wrote several books, but *Anticancer: A New Way of Life*[3] (Viking, 2009) was and is and, in my estimation, should remain a bestseller.

Another brilliant physician, Russell Blaylock, wrote a book that really focuses on the herbal/nutritional approach to cancer. *Natural Strategies for Cancer Patients*[4] (Kensington, 2003) is exquisitely readable and includes a very long list of references for his thinking—that is, all papers that have been published in the medical literature; the stuff that so many physicians call evidence that something might be helpful.

---

3 http://www.amazon.com/Anticancer-A-New-Way-Life/dp/0670021644

4 http://www.amazon.com/Natural-Strategies-Patients-Russell-Blaylock/dp/0758202210/ref=sr_1_1?s=books&ie=UTF8&qid=1383590950&sr=1-1&keywords=natural+strategies+for+cancer+patients+russell+blaylock+md

Doctors

The Institute for Functional Medicine is the best place to go to find an integrative or functional medical specialist.[1] Their web site's 'Find a Practitioner' service can help you to locate a practitioner anywhere in the world.

HeartMath

If you'd like to read more about HeartMath, I suggest starting with *The HeartMath Solution: The Institute of HeartMarth's Revolutionary Program for Engaging the Power of the Heart's Intelligence* (HarperCollins, 2011).[2]

Genetic Testing

BRACA testing is done through your oncologist or primary care doctor and is covered by insurance only if there is a family history that suggests genetics might be an issue in the maintenance of your health. For more detail on testing and how and when to go about doing it, resources are available at the Kimball Family Foundation.[3]

---

1 www.functionalmedicine.org

2 http://www.amazon.com/HeartMath-Solution-Rev-olutionary-Intelligence-ebook/dp/B004G8P2MS/ref=tmm_kin_swatch_0?_encoding=UTF8&sr=&qid=

3 http://www.kimballfamilyfoundation.com/index.shtml

Index

B

C

D

E

F

G

H

I

J

K

L

N

P

R

S

T

U

X

Y

Z

16297568R00315

Made in the USA
San Bernardino, CA
26 October 2014